ADVENTURES IN CREATIVE MOVEMENT ACTIVITIES

A Guide for Teaching

Second Edition

by

Marcia L. Lloyd, Ed.D.

Professor of Dance
Idaho State University

eddie bowers publishing, inc.

ACKNOWLEDGMENTS

I would like to extend my special love, thanks, and appreciation to the people who have helped me in this project:

To my husband, Arthur, who stayed at my side offering encouragement and providing invaluable assistance in proofreading and editing the final copies of both the first and second revised editions of this book.

To my children, Lisa and Arthur, Jr. for their encouragement, support, and belief in my work.

To all of my students at Idaho State University, the ISU Early Learning Center, the Cre-Act I School, Universiti Pertanian Malaysia, Universiti Malaya, Persatuan Tadika Malaysia, and the Classroom Teachers throughout the state of Idaho, all of whom, over the years have affirmed the value of creative movement and creative dance and the activities presented in this book.

To Connie C. Johnson for the cover photo.

Special thanks to Susan Duncan, Cheryle Lemmon, Randy Stamm, Thomas Stratton, and Al and Jane Strickland, for invaluable technical assistance provided for this second revised edition.

Marcia Lou Kemp Lloyd, Ed.D.
Professor of Dance
Idaho State University
December 1996

eddie bowers publishing, inc.
P.O. Box 130
Peosta, Iowa 52068-0130 USA

ISBN 0-945483-71-6

Copyright © 1998 by *eddie bowers publishing, inc.*

Printed in the United States of America.

9 8 7 6 5 4 3

CONTENTS

LIST OF FIGURES

PREFACE

During some of my early trips to Malaysia (1984, 1985, 1987, 1988, 1989), I conducted workshops in creative dance for practicing preschool/kindergarten teachers and taught courses in dance for education students at two universities. These workshops and courses were well received; and within a short time, I had reached thousands of teachers and students. While I was able to communicate most of my ideas through demonstration, dance, and extensive body language (since for many of the teachers and students, English was a second, third, or unknown language), I tried to prepare handouts for the courses whenever possible. As I met with groups of teachers and students throughout East and West Malaysia, however, the need became increasingly greater for an especially designed book in the area of creative dance for children—that could be a resource for these teachers when they were in their own classrooms.

Therefore, the English edition of *Adventures in Creative Movement Activities* was published in Malaysia in 1990 and a translated version with additional materials was published in the Malaysian language in 1994. Also a second printing in English with minor changes to the first edition was released in 1990. This printing, referred to as the international edition, was distributed in the United States by the National Dance Association and others and has been used by some universities for courses such as Creative Dance for Children and Methods and Techniques of Teaching Dance.

One of the strengths of *Adventures in Creative Movement Activities* has been the heavy emphasis on lessons and activities that can be used by classroom teachers from preschool through the university. By providing these practical activities in a logical, cookbook fashion, I believe that I have been faithful to those teachers and students in my early workshops and dance classes. They wanted something that they could use without extensive reading. Another strength of the book has been the underlying theory for creative dance that enables the teachers to go beyond using only the lessons in the book. As I began to consider this current revision, I believed that both the theory and practice areas of my book had proven, at least to me, that I should stay with this same combination of content—theory and application.

By the time that the inventory for the international version of the book had become quite low, I believed that the demand still existed for my book; therefore, I was very pleased when I was contacted by Eddie Bowers Publishing, Inc. with an opportunity for a revised edition.

In this new edition, I have thoroughly revised each chapter as needed, and have added a chapter on Creating Your Own Contemporary Folk Dance and a chapter discussing Assessment and Evaluation. Also, I have included a list of music, books, and video resources. Internet information for linking up with dance news groups, libraries, and the endless sources of information that are now accessible via the computer has been added. Further, I have added an appendix with additional lessons as a result of numerous requests from teachers, who in many cases were willing to provide samples of the lessons that they had created in their classes with their students.

In contacts with these same teachers, I was also encouraged to remain with the word *movement* in the title rather than *dance*. While I have been bonded to the word *dance* all of my professional life, I had originally substituted the word movement out of respect to many of my Malaysian students who were Muslims (a religion that seems to have reservations about the art of dance). As the book was used in the United States, however, I realized that the term *creative movement* also attracted readers who shied away from the term *creative dance*. Seemingly, some readers had an immediate reaction when they saw *dance* in the title of the book. They believed that, "Since I can't dance, this won't be useful for me in the classroom." So while definitions of creative movement and creative dance may differ somewhat, I have chosen the word *movement* for the title but have used *movement* and *dance* within the book to create a connection, hopefully, between the two.

Finally, as stated in the preface for the first edition, "This book is designed for teachers of all age groups from pre-school through university who wish to use creative movement activities in the classroom, gymnasium, or on the playground. These methods and techniques for training students in problem solving and decision making within creative movement activities can also be applied easily to other subject matter as well."

I HEAR AND I FORGET

I SEE AND I REMEMBER

I DO AND I UNDERSTAND

-PROVERB-

Chapter 1

THE FIRST STEP

INTRODUCTION

Creative movement should be an essential part of all levels of education. It is the basis for exploring our bodies and their capacities in preparation for sports, leisure activities, and healthy living. To the same extent that we want active, creative minds for our students, we should also want these minds to be housed in active, creative bodies.

This chapter introduces the beginning of the journey toward creating active minds and bodies by presenting definitions of creative dance, creative movement, a rationale for the inclusion of creative movement and dance in education, the objectives of creative movement, and the values of creative movement. Also presented in this chapter is background information about *enthusiastically* teaching creative movement activities and the vital role of the teacher in creative movement. The adventure now beings.

DEFINITION OF TERMS

Many definitions of creative dance and creative movement exist. A few definitions used by well known dance educators in the field have been presented here for teachers to ponder. Untimately, however, teachers must consider the commonalities of various definitions and then create their own interpretations, defining creative dance and creative movement for themselves and their students.

Creative Dance

Gilbert (1992) addressed this problem by stating that:

> . . . creative dance combines the mastery of movement with the artistry of expression. It is this combination, rather than a separation of the two, that makes creative dance so powerful. I have seen creative dance taught as merely an acquisition of dance skills on the one hand or unbridled expression on the other. I have also seen creative dance classes which consist solely of imitating nature or dancing stories or an activity in which only children too young to study "real" dance take part. I feel that when creative dance combines skill development and self-expression, it can be learned at any age level and enjoyed throughout a lifetime (p. 3).

Joyce (1994) considered the emotional and cultural qualities of creative dance when she stated that:

> Dance is so many things! It can be a leap for joy, a series of steps set to music, a religious ritual, or a work of art. It can be anything from the prance of mating pigeons to Pavlova's "dying swan."
>
> People dance socially. They dance to entertain. They also dance to communicate their deepest feelings. This is the goal of creative dance: *to communicate through movement* (p. 1).

Creative Movement

Creative movement, according to this author, is a unique form of self expression in which each participant uses rhythmic movements to express his or her thoughts, ideas, and/or feelings. The goal is to communicate through movement. Body, space, time and force (or energy) are the components of creative movement and are used as a basis for describing movement in this book. Creative movement (or creative dance) involves a process of the individual or the group selecting movements, sequencing the movements to express the theme, and performing the dance for self and/or others. Creative dance/movement is NOT a series of "steps" or "routines" taught by the teacher and imposed on the student. Rather, the movement patterns are created by the students with guidance from the teacher. Dunkin (1988) commented that:

We often speak of creative movement, a phrase which, for some people, conjures up a picture of simply turning on a record and handing the child a scarf with the instruction "dance to the music." Creative movement is an exploratory process which needs the same degree of consideration and preparation as any other dance course (p. 31).

Fleming (1976) concluded that, "problem solving, experimentation, discovery, taking chances, designing, taking [cues], making choices and judgments, [and] sharing relationships" are some of the opportunitities provided by creative movement experiences (p. 9).

Creativity

Humphrey (1987) stated that, "The word 'creative' derives from the Latin word *creatus*, one meaning of which is 'produced through imaginative skill.'" He stated that "The child should be given sufficient freedom to create his own responses in the situation he faces" (p. 40). He advocated the need for children to be involved in self-expressive activities, such as experimenting with ideas, expressing original ideas, thinking, and reacting. Humphrey (1987) further stated that, "Creativity and childhood enjoy a congruous relationship in that children are naturally creative. They imagine. They pretend. They are uninhibited. They are not only original but actually ingenious in their thoughts and actions" (p. 115).

Creativity is an important concept to consider in educating any age group. The child in all of us is full of curiosity and imagination and is uninhibited in movement expressions. These characteristics (curiosity, imagination, and being uninhibited) serve as an excellent foundation for providing creative movement experiences that will assist students of all ages to further develop the unique individuals that they are.

Everyone possesses a degree of creativity—a unique gift used for self expression. When comparing ourselves with others, though, we may not believe that we are creative. This type of comparison is unfair, however, because each person's creativity is nurtured and developed in many different ways. When applying the following definition of creativity to ourselves, each one of us will find, though, that he or she has participated in one or more of the aspects listed—concluding that everyone is creative to a certain extent. Murray (1975) quoted June King McFee as stating that:

"Creativity". . . refers to people's behavior when they do such things as (1) invent a new pattern, form, or idea; (2) rearrange already established objects, patterns, or ideas; and (3) integrate a new or borrowed factor into an already established organization (p. 27).

Based on this definition of creativity, and the idea that creativity involves inventiveness and productivity, teachers need to examine the extent to which creative experiences are being offered in their schools and answer the following questions:

1. What creative experience activities are present in my school and classroom?

2. Are these activities cultivated, nurtured, and encouraged?

3. How are the students being aided in developing creative potential?

Murray (1975) stressed the value of the arts in the development of the child's personality when she cited Lydia Joel as stating that:

To a child the arts are not play, they are meaningful work. They are ways of saying how he feels and who he is. And if the curiosity and eagerness the arts stir in him are turned off . . . by boredom, lack of involvement, or insensitive adults . . . the fragile structure of ego built upon confidence in his capacity to make judgments, to risk failure, to try and try again until he is satisfied . . . will shrink, hide, and sometimes collapse. It needs support in the form of gentle guidance and respect (p. 27).

Teachers play a major role in helping students develop creative potential. Helping students explore, discover, and develop the gift of creativity is quite possibly the most exciting adventure upon which a teacher can embark. The following seven comments provide "food for thought" about creativity, creative movement, and creative dance:

1. Creativity is the one type of giftedness that is found to some degree in all students but that is often stifled by the restrictive classroom environments.

2. Creativity is a natural way of learning. It is both personal and fun and all students can be successful in their own way.

3. Creativity cannot be left to chance. Dance can provide the schools the means by which children can succeed, by posing problems with open-ended responses.

(continued)

4. Dance involves little expense for creative experiences because it is self-contained.

5. Creative dance offers the students another way to see themselves as truly unique individuals because there are no ready-made answers on how to feel, see, think, or move their bodies through space.

6. Students develop their own creative capacities and learn to relate openly and cooperatively with others through the emotional, mental and physical demands of dance.

7. Creative dance requires the students to inquire, think, sense, observe, feel, invent, respond, and to evaluate. During this process the teacher should be a guide, not impose set movements and feelings upon the students. As skills evolve through the creative process, they can later be applied to the traditional patterns and compositions introduced by the teacher. (*Dance: A Guide for Idaho Public Schools. Grades K-12*, 1991, p. 6)

Many terms suitably describe the process of creating movement for self expressive purposes. Terms such as creative movement, creative dance, creative rhythmic movement, rhythms, rhythmic activities, or creative movement activities are all used. The idea, however, is not to be overly concerned with terms. The main idea is to develop movement activities that encourage the growth and development of creative potential in students. The use of appropriate terms along with a careful introduction of new activities, however, might win support from community groups which would otherwise not be as accepting of movement activities.

RATIONALE FOR THE INCLUSION OF CREATIVE MOVEMENT AND DANCE IN EDUCATION

"Dance education is a medium for enhancing the quality of life for children, youth, and adults. Every human being has the right to move in ways that are primal, expressive, imaginative, and transformational" (*Dance as Education*, p. 45). Creative movement should be an essential part of all levels of education. It is the basis for exploring our bodies and their capacities in preparation for sports, leisure activities, and healthy living. As stated earlier, to the same extent that we want active, creative minds for our students, we should also want these minds to be housed in active, creative bodies.

Purcell (1994) makes a strong case for the significant role that dance can play in the curriculum when she stated that:

> Dance should be an integral component of a comprehensive education for the same reasons that math, history, language arts, social studies, the arts, and science are essential to education. The body of knowledge in each subject area teaches children who they are and how they interact with the world—past, present, and future. The unique aspect of dance that makes its inclusion in the elementary curriculum imperative is that dance fully integrates the cognitive, motor, and affective domains within each task. Children simultaneously move, think, and feel. In no other subject area do children learn to communicate and express themselves through movement, a natural means of expression for children. Through dance, children can learn history, music, visual arts, theater, language arts, science, math, social studies, and health. They learn about themselves and how they relate to others and the world as moving, thinking, feeling human beings (p. vii).

Bennett and Riemer (1995) prefaced their book with the following comments concerning the importance of dance:

> "To dance is to live and to live is to dance," according to Snoopy in the *Peanuts* comic strip. We have both spent our entire adult lives (and many of our childhood years) dancing to live and living to dance. . . . Possibly the greatest antidote to aging is physical activity. Dance can rejuvenate almost anyone. . . . Dance offers a point of entry for students of all skill levels; dance is age appropriate and individually appropriate (p.v).

Gardner (1983) developed the Theory of Multiple Intelligences that offers an excellent rationale for the inclusion of creative dance and creative movement experiences in the school curriculum. Stinson (1991) cites him as theorizing that human beings possess seven different forms of knowing that include: "language, logic and mathematics, music, spatial information, bodily-kinesthetic information, knowledge about other persons (interpersonal), and knowledge about oneself (intrapersonal)" (pp. 51-52). Gardner (1983) also provides in his book information specifically about dance and its relationship to at least one of the intelligences in Chapter 9, Bodily-Kinesthetic Intelligence.

Since the Theory of Multiple Intelligences was first introduced, dance educators have been exploring the ways in which dance uses each one of these intelligences. In fact, perhaps more than any other discipline, creative dance and creative movement seem to employ all seven of these intelligences. A conference held in 1995 by the Dance Educators Association of Washington (DEAW) focused on exploring each one of the intelligences using 50-minute lessons taught by experts in the field of each intelligence. The participants truly experienced the theme of the conference which was "Moving Through The Multiple Intelligences." Further studies of the Theory of Multiple Intelligences and its connection to dance need to be conducted to provide additional evidence of the value this theory provides to teachers of all subjects including dance.

Rights of Children

Fleming (1976) suggested that movement and children are synonymous, and that thinking about one without the other is difficult. She stated that "Movement is a universal language of boys and girls, who use it to express reactions to us, to each other, to their world, to situations, and to things" (p. 4). Our first form of communication is through movement, well before birth. Each child is a unique individual, however, and has his or her own way of expressing feelings through movement. Therefore, each child should have the opportunity as a part of early school experiences to develop skills in the area of expressing himself or herself through movement.

The topic of human rights seems to be a major concern in the world today. Children, however, are often forgotten when considering the rights of individuals. In response to this void, Fleming (1976) provided a "Bill of Rights" for children. Teachers who have participated in workshops, seminars, and courses conducted by this author have enthusiastically copied Fleming's statement; consequently, the *"Bill of Rights"* is included in this book.

Bill of Rights

Let me grow as I be
And try to understand why I want to grow like me;
Not like my Mom wants me to be,
Nor like my Dad hopes I'll be
Or my teacher thinks I should be.
Please try to understand and help me grow
Just like me!
   (Fleming, 1976, p. 3)

How do we help students grow to be like themselves? Teachers have a tremendous responsibility to help students grow and develop as individuals. Teachers are obligated to offer their students opportunities to create and express themselves, and to accept these offerings from the students.

Developing a program of creative movement activities is not a small task, especially with a classroom full of busy, active students who may have short attention spans and high energy levels that often exceed those of the teacher. This book has been written to assist the teacher in channeling that energy and in developing a creative movement activity program that will offer students opportunities to experience self expression through movement.

OBJECTIVES OF CREATIVE MOVEMENT

The goal to have creative movement as a part of the education for children seems to exist in many cultures around the world. And in fact, the teaching of creative movement is frequently associated with the teaching of cultural appreciation. An example of one country's attempt to address creative movement activities was outlined in a seminar paper, *Pre-School Curriculum Guidelines for Malaysia,* in which the rapid growth and development of pre-school education was discussed. Nine general objectives and a set of specific objectives for each area were listed in the paper. The ninth general objective, *The Development of Aesthetic Appreciation and Creativity,* stated that:

Children are naturally (basically) creative. During the preschool years, they are not only able to express their thoughts and feelings effectively through language, but feelings of happiness, anger, sadness, fear and disappointment which they experience can also be expressed through art and craft, music and movement. Given proper guidance by the teacher, these children will be encouraged to demonstrate their imaginativeness and creativity in a variety of ways using a variety of materials.

Specific Objectives

1. To express feelings through art and craft, music and movement;

2. To experiment using a variety of materials to create something;

3. To listen to and enjoy music and to participate in music and movement activities;

4. To develop (nurture) creativity through art and craft, music and movement activities;

5. To sing and enjoy simple songs;

6. To know and appreciate the cultures of diverse ethnic groups in Malaysia (1972, p. 12).

Creative movement activities are certainly one way to achieve the objectives listed above. This list, however, when compared with educational goals in the United States would also be very adaptable to the education of American children. In a similar vein, the National Standards for Arts Education (1994) provide a series of content standards and achievement standards for students in American schools from kindergarten through grade 12 in dance, music, theatre, and visual arts. These goals for dance include the understanding, creating, performing, and appreciating of dance. See Chapter 12 for further information pertaining to these national standards for dance.

VALUES OF CREATIVE MOVEMENT

Creative movement activities provide many values to the participants. Ayob (1986) conducted a study entitled, "An Examination of Purpose Concepts in Creative Dance For Children," in which she stated:

> Creative dance for children which deals with the psychomotor, the affective, and the cognitive domains of human learning is of particular value to all children. It promotes the understanding of the communicative and expressive nature of movement. It stimulates divergent and critical thinking, imagination, creativity and problem solving . . . (p. ii).

Ayob (1986) confirmed that creative dance not only contributes to general educational values but specifically to the three domains in which children are educated: the cognitive (mind), the psychomotor (body), and the affective (attitudes and appreciation). Bennett and Riemer (1995) have also identified characteristics that apply to each one of these three domains in order to enhance lesson planning and to ultimately assess the achievements of students. See Chapter 12 for their contributions.

An additional value provided by creative movement is that it is a success-oriented activity for everyone for the following reasons:

1. It allows the student to proceed at his or her own rate.

2. The student's solution to the movement problem is accepted by the teacher.

3. It builds a positive self-concept in the student as a result of the first two reasons.

Joyce (1980) suggested that creative dance is unique and provides valuable experiences that no other discipline offers.

It is the only activity in which physical movement is used nonfunctionally and as a personal expression. Children find a fulfillment through dance that can be realized through no other discipline, because dance simultaneously involves the inner being and the physical body. In dancing, children are not concerned with a game, an object, or even another person; their concentration and awareness are fixed on the act of moving.

Because of this focus, children discover a great deal about their bodies, minds, language, thoughts, imagination, and ideas through creative dance. . . . Dance experience teaches children both awareness and control of movement. They use these skills in games, sports, and everyday living. . . . Movement as creative expression plays an important part in life, building self-image, self-awareness, and self-direction. . . . It is a clearly defined body of knowledge, in that it deals with elements that can be explored, learned, managed, and used. In other words, creative dance is a discipline for dealing with the self (pp. 4-5).

Stinson (1988) indicated several values of creative movement experiences for children. She said it "is concerned with sensory awareness of movement and deep involvement in the experience" (p. 4). Developing sensory awareness is a valuable skill for young children to learn, as is the development of kinesthetic awareness (awareness of muscle movement). Stinson (1988) also suggested that creative movement experiences can teach children personal joy and fulfillment through the arts (rather than drugs). She stated that creative movement experiences can help children learn ". . . how to find meaning and exhilaration in activities that will nourish them rather than destroy them" (p. 8-9).

Other values that creative movement experiences can provide for students and teachers are ways of:

1. Creating an overall education by understanding the culture and heritage of self and others,

2. Solving complex and difficult problems,

(continued)

3. Developing and enlarging movement vocabulary,

4. Providing cognitive learning experiences,

5. Assuming responsibility for one's own choices,

6. Learning to concentrate and focus attention, and

7. Developing awareness of and respect for others.

Creative movement experiences can also provide a value that is akin to survival. In a society that some believe is becoming more violent and inhumane, creative movement offers the opportunity for young people to "dance out their fears and feelings" in a safe environment. One example of this is provided by Soundance, a dance company that was formed in 1985. As part of its community commitment, Sandra Stratton, artistic director, has offered dance and drama workshops for children six years through adolescence at a junior high school in the Lower East Side of New York City (referred to as the second city). The number of students participating in the program swelled from twelve in the first class in 1985 to more than fifty (ages 8-18) in 1994. An annual theme is selected and teachers, students, and artists collaborate on creating a presentation. "Stratton points out that such a process ensures that 'we're almost always dealing with the life issues that they're dealing with. If it's not violence, it's sexuality or it's drugs' " (Tobias, 1994, p. 78). One important value that creative dance offers these children from an inner city environment is illustrated by the following:

Each year, during the Soundance workshop, a number of young people set out to learn how to work together and often, on the way, discover what it means to take responsiblity for themselves. Through dancing and acting, they find their voices and begin to understand how to articulate their own concerns and those of their peers. In concluding the dramatic scene about their schoolmate's death [stabbed to death at school], the performers in last year's workshop asked, "Who's going to stop the violence?" And then, in answer: "We are—and"—pointing at the crowd of children in the audience—"you." Creative expression may yet transform the second city (Tobias, 1994, p. 79).

CONTENT OF THE BOOK

This book is designed to provide teachers with a specific approach to immediately begin teaching creative   movement to their students.The material is intended to be practical, useful, and easy to present.

The sample lessons have been taught successfully to students of various cultures, age groups, and abilities, including preschool through older adults. The teachers who have tested the ideas contained in the sample lessons have reported immediate success. Also, ways to create, develop, and extend lessons are suggested; and additional lessons created by teachers and students are included in an appendix at the end of the book.

AN ENTHUSIASTIC BEGINNING

Teachers do not need to have previous training in physical education or movement-activity experiences in order to succeed in teaching creative movement to their students. What the teacher does need is an "I CAN SUCCEED" attitude and the courage to take the "first step." A philosopher once suggested that a journey of a thousand miles begins with the first step. The most difficult part of any task or adventure is the beginning. Previous experiences with teachers in various countries have shown that courage and enthusiasm are already present in the behaviors of classroom teachers and all that is needed is a way to begin. This book provides an easy way to begin teaching creative movement and opens many new doors for teachers and their students.

OPENING NEW DOORS

As encouragement to teachers new to the concept of teaching creative movement, the author will share one of the experiences she had while conducting workshops for teachers in Malaysia. Although this example occurred in Southeast Asia, she has had similar experiences on numerous occasions with teachers in other countries and several of the states in the United States.

In late 1987, a group of 25 preschool teachers met in Kuala Lumpur for two hours each week over a period of five weeks to learn techniques for teaching creative movement activities and to develop a lesson each week to share with their students. During the days following each workshop session, the teachers presented that lesson to their students and returned the next week to share the results with the workshop group. Only a few of these teachers possessed previous training or experience in dance or physical education; yet, **all** of the teachers reported a successful experience with their students each week.

All of the teachers were surprised and amazed that even the first creative movement lesson they taught was a success for the students and for themselves. The teachers reported that the students were actually begging for more creative movement experiences. Several teachers reported that during the recess time they had observed the students doing the same movement activity which had been taught that day. In fact, one teacher observed several students grouped together creating new movements which they added to the pattern that they had learned earlier.

Instant success for the teachers and the students came with their very first movement experience together. All that was needed for successful creative movement experiences was a way to start opening doors to new ideas.

Success, however, does have a formula. Part of the plan for success is provided in this book, and the other part of the plan comes from the courage and enthusiasm of the teacher. This book's contribution to the formula deals with presenting the philosophy and processes of movement and conveying the understanding that creative movement is a success-oriented activity for all of the students. Creative movement activities are based on the students' individual responses being accepted by the teacher. The following statements about creative dance and creative movement are important to remember:

1. There is no wrong way to move.

2. The only competition is within oneself.

3. There are no losers in creative movement activities.

4. Every student (and every teacher) is a winner with creative movement.

THE ROLE OF THE TEACHER

The teacher's role in creative movement is to guide the students in the process of creating and expressing thoughts, ideas and/or feelings through movement, and to facilitate (or make easier) varied movement experiences. In creative movement, then, the teacher does not teach steps to be memorized; instead, the teacher helps the students explore many different kinds of movement in as many ways as possible.

In teaching, according to Joyce (1994), "you seek to reach the part of the individual that is a composer rather than a player, an originator rather than an interpreter, a creator rather than a performer" (p. 1). She continued with the idea that, "The need to move makes children improve their ability to move. The teacher's role is to keep challenging them to stimulate and fulfill this need. The overall purpose is to open up movement as a means of expression" (pp. 5-6). The most important thing to remember about creative movement is that the **process** is more important than the product; the experience of creating movement can be an end in itself.

SUMMARY

Creative movement is a unique form of self expression in which each participant selects movements to express his or her thoughts, ideas, or feelings. Creative movement is to be experienced, it is not a series of "steps" or "routines" taught by the teacher.

Creative movement activity contains many values for students of all ages and abilities, as well as for teachers, because it provides a new way to learn and teach. Some of these values include developing a movement vocabulary, increasing movement skills, learning to solve movement problems, understanding one's own and others' cultures, and expanding learning in the cognitive, psychomotor, and affective domains.

Through creative movement and dance, students develop body awareness, a positive self-concept, and a new relationship with self and others. In doing so, creative movement activities seem to provide the means to achieve many of the specific objectives of the school curriculum. Creative movement activities also provide an avenue of socially acceptable expression for children from environments where free expression is inhibited and models for appropriate expression are limited.

Gardner's (1983) Theory of Multiple Intelligences challenges teachers to consider a variety of ways of learning and teaching.

Teachers need no previous training in movement activities. What they do need is enthusiasm, courage, and an "I CAN SUCCEED" attitude to take the first step in teaching creative movement. The role of the teacher is to serve as a guide or facilitator in helping students explore, experiment, and discover ways of moving that can serve as a means of self expression. The teacher then accepts these movement responses as a natural part of the development of the students.

Chapter 2

COMPONENTS
OF
CREATIVE MOVEMENT

INTRODUCTION

All physical activity involves the elements of body, time, space, and force. These elements, which are used automatically in everyday activities, are also the foundation used to build creative movement and creative dance experiences.

None of the elements operate independently, but the teacher can select and emphasize one element at a time for teaching purposes. This procedure helps direct and limit the goals of a lesson. By recognizing ways to select individual movement topics, the teacher who is new to the instruction of creative movement activities will not be overwhelmed by too many elements at one time. What becomes marvelously overwhelming, however, is reaching the point when the teacher and students discover after only a few lessons the never-ending movement combinations these elements provide.

This chapter introduces the elements of creative movement, the fundamental movements, and ways to develop a series of creative movement activities.

ELEMENTS OF CREATIVE MOVEMENT

As stated, the elements of movement include body, time, space, and force. Some educators consider flow as a separate element, but in this book, flow will be merged with force and will be defined in relationship to this fourth element.

Body

The body is the instrument or tool used to express an idea, thought, or feeling. The body can be divided into the following two categories (based partially on Joyce, 1980, pp. 4-5):

Inner parts of the body, such as the heart, lungs, and other organs, which are in constant motion and operate most of the time without our conscious awareness (involuntary movements).

Outer parts of the body, such as the head, shoulders, arms, hands, fingers, torso, legs, feet, and toes, which usually take some conscious effort to move (voluntary movements).

Movement ideas are expressed by use of body parts, surfaces (front, back, sides), and shapes formed by the body.

Time

Time "properties" include all of the various ways that emphasis and duration are measured or observed in creative movement. Time is delineated in the following ways:

Tempo	— how fast or slow the movement is performed
Beat	— the continuous sound of the underlying rhythm—like a heart beat
Accent	— a stronger beat within a rhythmic pattern
Duration	— the length of each beat or pattern
Rhythmic Patterns —	a combination of tempo, beat, accent, and duration

Space

Space is concerned with two general dimensions and a set of spatial elements. These elements are expressed in the following descriptions:

Personal Space (or **Self Space**) extends in any direction as far as an individual can bend, stretch, or reach.

General (or **Environmental Space**) includes the classroom, gymnasium, or playground where movement activities take place.

(continued)

Spatial elements include:

Direction — forward, sideward, backward, diagonal

Level — high, medium, low

Range — near, far,

Size — big, little

Pathway — curved, straight, angular

Shape — narrow, wide, angular, circular, straight

Focus — the direction in which the eyes are looking.

Force

Force is used in every movement and is categorized in terms of weak to strong, sharp to smooth, and heavy to light. The amount of energy expended in a movement demonstrates force or lack of force. According to Joyce (1980) "All movement can be altered by changes in force, depending on the *attack* (sharp or smooth), the *weight* (heavy or light), the *strength* (tight or loose), and the *flow* (free flowing, bound, or in balance)" (p. 4).

Flow

Flow is connected with force because of the use of energy when movement occurs. The body is either free flowing, bound, or in balance.

Free flowing — movements are continuous, ongoing, and fluid. Stopping is difficult with free flowing movements.

Bound — movements are controlled, balanced, and restrained. Stopping is easy with bound movements.

Balance — indicates a position that is located between free flowing movement and bound movement.

FUNDAMENTAL MOVEMENTS

Fundamental movements of the body in motion include nonlocomotor and locomotor actions.

Nonlocomotor Movements

Nonlocomotor movements are performed on a stationary base. The person is standing or sitting in one place. These are also known as axial movements because the movements are performed around the axis of the body. Examples of nonlocomotor movements are as follows:

Bending	— bringing body parts closer together
Stretching	— full extension of any body part
Twisting	— rotation of a part of the body; or the whole body
Turning	— rotation of the whole body
Rising	— moving the body from a lower to a higher position (such as from lying on the floor, to sitting, to kneeling, to standing)
Falling	— moving the body from a higher position to a lower position
Swinging	— moving a part of the body in an arc or circle
Pushing	— moving a body part (or prop) away from the body center
Pulling	— moving a body part (or prop) toward the body center

Locomotor Movements

Locomotor movements are performed on a moving base and take the body through space from one place to another. The cited portions of the following definitions were taken from the glossary in Harris, Pittman, and Waller (1994).

Even rhythmic patterns:

Walking — "steps from one foot to the other, the weight being transferred from heel to toe" (p. 523). The movement emphasis is mainly directional.

Running — "similar to [walking], except that the weight is carried forward over the ball of the foot with a spring-like action" (p. 519). The movement emphasis becomes one of a faster tempo than walking.

Leaping — "a transfer of weight from one foot to the other foot. Push off with a spring and land on the ball of the other foot, letting the heel come down; bend the knee to absorb the shock" (p. 515). The movement emphasis is up and over.

Jumping — "one or both feet leave the floor, knees bending; both return to the floor together, landing toe-heel with an easy knee action to catch body weight. Spring off the floor on the upbeat of the music and land on the beat" (p. 515). The movement emphasis is upward.

Hopping — "a transfer of weight by a springing action from one foot to the same foot" (p. 515). The movement emphasis is upward.

Uneven rhythmic patterns:

Skipping — "a step and a hop on the same foot in slow quick slow quick rhythm" (p.520); alternate feet. The movement emphasis is upward.

Galloping — "moving forward diagonally with a step close step close pattern (slow, quick, slow, quick)" (p. 514); the same foot leads each pattern, the other foot follows. The movement emphasis is downward.

Sliding — "is a step close step close pattern (slow, quick, slow, quick)" (p. 520); the same foot leads each pattern, the other foot follows; movement performed to the right or left side. The movement emphasis is usually sideward.

Locomotor movements can be also divided into the following even or uneven rhythmic patterns:

Even rhythmic patterns are performed to a steady, regular beat (each beat lasting the same length of time). The pattern can be counted (such as 1-2-3-4) and notated as appears in Figure 1. The even rhythmic pattern could be for a walk, run, hop, leap, jump, or a combination of any of these movements. The even rhythmic pattern illustrated in Figure 1 depicts a walk.

Uneven rhythmic patterns combine a long beat with a short beat. The notation for an uneven pattern will appear in written form as: 1 & 2 & 3 & 4 &, with the number being the long beat and the "&" (and) being the short beat. The uneven pattern could be for a skip, slide, gallop, or any combination of these movements. The uneven rhythmic pattern illustrated in Figure 1 is for a skip. Each pattern illustrated shows one measure (or unit) of 4 beats.

Examples of Even and Uneven Rhythmic Patterns

___1___	A long beat which receives one full count. A series of long beats results in an even rhythmic pattern.		
__1__ __&__	A beat of "1" (approximately 3/4 of a long beat) and a short beat of "&" (approximately 1/4 of a long beat) together result in an uneven pattern the length of one full beat.		

Even	Step	Step	Step	Step
(walk)	1	2	3	4
Uneven	Step hop	Step hop	Step hop	Step hop
(skip)	1 &	2 &	3 &	4 &

A measure can contain any number of beats depending on the pattern required. Most measures consist of two, three, four, six, or eight beats. When several measures are combined, a phrase of music or movement is the result.

Figure 1.

Remember that in the *uneven* rhythmic pattern in Figure 1, the duration of the long beat and the short beat combined equals the duration of one beat in the *even* rhythmic pattern.

DEVELOPING A SERIES OF CREATIVE MOVEMENT ACTIVITIES

One way to begin developing a series of creative movement lessons is to explore each one of the elements (body, time, space, or force) separately, although all of the elements work in combination with each other. Start with one simple idea. For example: explore how many different ways one body part, such as the arm, can move. Begin by asking the students questions like:

1. How many different directions can you move one arm?

2. How fast (or slow) can one arm move?

3. Can you make that same arm swing forward, backward, and in a circle?

4. Now can you try moving your other arm fast and then slow, and swing it forward, backward, and in a circle?

In this list of questions, the arm was the main body element to be explored, while the elements of space (directions in which the arm can move), time (fast and slow), and force (the energy expended in swinging the arm, such as using a great deal of energy to begin the swinging and very little energy to end the swinging movement) were also explored.

Expand this activity by adding another body part such as a leg, knee, or foot. Explore the movement of body parts individually and then in combination. The addition of other elements will continually challenge the creative potential of both the teacher and the students and keep the movement activity fresh and alive.

By combining nonlocomotor movements with locomotor movements, a rhythmic pattern can be created and eventually evolve into a movement composition. For example, a basic pattern can be created that combines the following movements: 4 walks, 2 stretches, 2 bends and stretches, 4 hops, one twist, and one turn.

A number of decisions must be made as a movement pattern is created. Problems must be solved concerning the use of the body, space, time, and force. The students can make many of the choices either as a group or individually. The teacher can begin by making suggestions and then allowing the students to create their own ways of performing the pattern. Here is one way to begin and the words a teacher can use:

1. Everyone take 4 walking steps forward around your own circle.

2. Stop and stretch one arm very slowly, then stretch the other arm very slowly.

3. Bend and stretch one knee very fast; bend and stretch one elbow very fast.

4. Hop 4 times in any direction you choose, without bumping into anyone.

5. Stop and twist your whole body into a very low shape. Hold that shape so that everyone can look at all of the low shapes in the room.

6. Take one full turn of the body and freeze in place.

This pattern can be practiced a few times until the students are familiar with the movements and then can be changed or extended in the following ways:

1. Repeat the entire pattern twice in exactly the same way.

2. Perform the pattern in the order in which it appears, then perform the pattern in reverse order.

3. Mix the order of the pattern.

4. Allow the students to suggest changes in the pattern.

Another way to plan creative movement patterns is to draw upon the basic questions of What? Where? With Whom or With What? and How? Make a chart that is divided into four boxes. (See Figures 7 and 8 in Chapter Eight for examples of this chart.) The squares in the chart can be filled in by the teacher with suggestions from the students, or by the students themselves after the first experience.

The chart can be made any size, but using poster paper or a chalkboard would be better for classroom use. An overhead transparency can be used multiple times as long as "washable" marking pens are used. Each square can be represented by a color on any visual aid created. Suggestions for colors appear in parentheses at the end of each statement. The students may wish to select their own color code.

In each quarter of the chart, the teacher and students should supply answers to the following:

1. **What is to be moved?** This addresses body awareness as the students consider the various body parts and shapes. (Red)

2. **Where is the body or body part to be moved?** This addresses personal and environmental awareness of space, and introduces directions, levels, and pathways. (Blue)

3. **With Whom or With What are the students to move?**

   With Whom? This introduces relationship awareness as the students consider individuals versus pairs versus groups.

   With What? This introduces how body parts relate to one another and what parts may be moved together, and/or objects which may be introduced as props in the movement activity. (Green)

4. **How are the body parts or students to move?** This addresses awareness of time (tempo, beat, accent, duration) and force (expenditure of energy). (Orange)

By making selections from each of the four areas of awareness, a pattern of creative movement will develop. Colors can be used to indicate the body, space, ti\me/force, and relationships of with whom or with what as suggested in the figure illustrating the four areas.

SUMMARY

This chapter presented the components of creative movement (the elements of body, time, space, and force) and the fundamental movements (nonlocomotor and locomotor). Ways to combine movements were also suggested, and a beginning movement pattern that used nonlocomotor movements (bending, stretching, twisting, and turning) and locomotor movements (walking and hopping) was presented.

The teacher and students, however, will want to consider the wide variety of elements and fundamental movements described in the following chapters to create more movement activities that will further challenge and expand their skills and abilities.

Chapter **3**

STRUCTURE OF CREATIVE MOVEMENT LESSONS

INTRODUCTION

Creative movement experiences do not happen without careful planning and organization by the teacher. According to Russell (1968), each lesson should have a primary emphasis and also "should aim to provide opportunities for the child to develop an understanding of his own movement capacities, to learn the language of movement and so invent and create sequences and dances of his own" (p. 17). She stated further that, "In the primary school we should aim to increase the child's power of observation and his sensitive awareness to movement, sound, shape, texture and rhythm" (p.18).

To provide these and other opportunities, objectives for each unit and lesson plan should be clearly specified and continually evaluated as the creative process occurs. A unit usually involves several lesson plans, each plan is designed to be presented for one period of time such as 30 minutes as illustrated in this book. Each lesson plan should build upon the previous plan to further explore the selected theme.

Creative movement experiences usually begin with selecting a theme or movement topic and creating lesson plans that explore this topic. Sometimes, however, an idea for a single lesson occurs and then a theme or topic evolves around which the teacher can build a unit. This text provides units of movement (body, time, space, and force) with two lessons already developed. Other themes, movement topics, or single lessons can be designed to explore movement or dance in areas such as language arts, mathematics, geography, history, science, cultural studies, literature, and other curricular areas.

This chapter provides guidelines designed to assist the teacher in developing and teaching enjoyable, exciting, and successful creative movement lessons. To accomplish this, a format for developing lessons is presented, and an example of a lesson plan form is included at the end of the chapter. An extra set of the eight lesson plans that were written for this book (in Chapters 4-7) along with additional blank lesson plan forms (to write your own lessons) are provided in an appendix at the end of the book. Also included in an appendix are lessons created by classroom teachers. These lessons can be used as they are or can serve as stimuli for further creative movement activities. Most of these lessons have some feedback by the teacher in the evaluation section of the lesson.

Recommendations are also offered in this chapter that teachers can use to establish an organized, yet free, atmosphere where students are allowed to create. The space to be used to conduct movement activities is also discussed. Finally, ideas are given for different types of accompaniment that can be used for creative movement activities.

FORMAT FOR A LESSON

The lessons in this book have been structured using a consistent format. This format has been used successfully to prepare creative movement lessons outlining experiences of 25 to 30 minutes for a classroom setting. The format begins with specific objectives and divides the creative movement activity into four parts: warm ups, movement exploration activities, a gathering activity (to culminate the lesson), and relaxation.

Lesson Plan Format

Objectives - Specific objectives should be created for each lesson. As the teacher gains additional experience in planning and teaching the lessons, the value of stating specific objectives for each lesson will become clear.

Warm-Ups *(about 5 minutes)* - A warming-up period provides the students with immediate activity such as gentle stretching and bending, twisting and turning (or other nonlocomotor movements); and walking, running, sliding, and skipping (or other locomotor movements). Each warm up should include both nonlocomotor and locomotor movements. The purpose of warm ups is to capture the students' attention and concentration and prepare them mentally and physically for the lesson.

Movement Exploration Activities (5-7 *minutes*) - The "movement topic-of-the-day" is introduced so that the students, with guidance from the teacher, can explore movement activities that focus on a central theme or topic. An introduction to the movement activity can be made in a variety of ways. Some of these ways include:

1. Use questions and challenges to introduce movement activities. To help the students explore movements of body parts, the teacher can pose questions such as:

    How many different ways can you move your arm?

    Can you show me a shape that you can make with both arms?

    Can you move one arm forward as you move the other backward?

2. Show a picture and briefly discuss various aspects of it, such as the colors, shapes of the objects, lines that are used, subject(s) of the picture, and actions in the picture. Select one aspect at a time and discuss how students could move to express this aspect, and then explore the movement ideas that were discussed.

3. Select appropriate music, or other accompaniment, that reflects the movement topic-of-the-day to assist the students in expressing themselves.

These three ways of introducing movement activities will challenge the imagination of both the teacher and the students and will help them discover many innovative ways of introducing and carrying out the lessons that are developed. The purpose of movement exploration is to have students begin to think about and perform the initial movement activities that are planned for the day.

Gathering Activity (*10-15 minutes*) - The gathering activity is the culmination of the lesson. The gathering activity brings together the lesson parts into one, peak experience.

When the students have explored the movement possibilities of the movement topic or theme for the lesson, they should be directed to select movements that show (or demonstrate) a beginning, a middle, and an ending of a movement pattern. The teacher guides the students in this phase of the lesson by making comments such as :

Let me see your starting shape.

What movement will you choose for the middle part of your pattern?

Can you show me your ending shape?

The teacher will then help the students put all of the movements together into a basic sequence of shape-movement-shape as follows:

1. A beginning shape (a stationary position),

2. A locomotor movement selected from the movement exploration activity, and

3. An ending shape (a stationary position).

As a way to begin the gathering activity, the teacher can use four counts for each part. (For ease of reading and counting, numerals have been used instead of writing out the word for the number of counts.) For example, the teacher can allow **4** counts to make a shape, **4** counts to move (walk, run, or another locomotor movement), and **4** counts to make another shape.

After a few experiences, the teacher can involve the students in decisions of *what kind of movements* they want to perform, *how long* (how many counts or beats) each part should be, *how much force* (or energy) should be used for each part, and the *amount of space* that will be needed for each part. Together, the teacher and students can plan ways to rearrange the movements such as starting with the ending shape, retaining the middle portion, and ending with what was previously the beginning shape. This gathering activity (or culminating experience) should bring all of the lesson parts together for a whole experience. It should give the movement form (a beginning, a middle, and an ending) and provide an opportunity for the students to create a sequence of movements within the basic structure provided.

As part of the gathering activity the teacher can provide a "**show-and-share**" time. This is a time set aside to provide individuals or groups of students with the opportunity to perform and observe the creative movement pieces that have been planned. "Show and share" can accomplish the tasks of preparing students to be part of an audience and prepare them to be performers. By dividing the class in half, one group can perform and the other group can watch. Then the groups can trade places. Through this process, the students begin learning the audience skills of observing quietly and attentively; and they can learn how to show appreciation by applauding at the proper time, as the performers take their bows. Performance skills develop as the students learn to follow the cues given for the proper time to begin the performance and learn how long to hold their ending shape so that the audience will sense when the piece is finished.

Another way to conduct a show-and-share experience is to allow each student to perform a movement of his or her choice, or to demonstrate the movement-of-the-day for the teacher. Joyce (1980) suggested a good-bye dance as a way to culminate the day's activity.

> . . . the children line up at the far side of the room and dance [one student at a time] to the teacher in any way they wish, as long as they include the element of the day. They must use the space of the room as much as possible and not simply dance in a straight path. They may dance as long as they wish, but must end with a shape. As each one finishes, he or she comes to sit beside the teacher, and the next in line begins (p. 48).

In reference to the *good-bye dance,* Joyce (1980) discovered that she never needed to be concerned about which child should begin. She stated that:

> There always seem to be some children who like to be first and some who like to be last, so lining up does not create trouble. You can start having the children do good-bye dances very early in the term, even on the first day. That first time they may just walk from their places in line to where you are sitting on the floor; they will make a shape and sit down next to you. Any child can do this, and it means that for a minute you are looking only at that child (pp. 48 & 51).

After the first few experiences with the *good-bye dance,* Joyce (1980) suggested that the teacher can ask each student, "How else can you walk to me?" (p. 51). The teacher can then watch to see the variety of ways of walking the students choose to show. They may walk in their regular way, backwards, diagonally, in a circle, or a new way.

In summary, the purpose of the gathering activity is to pull the lesson parts together into a form that contains a beginning, a middle, and an ending. Using this format, students create pieces that express the day's movement experiences. This activity also allows the students to see the movement achievement of others. The *good-bye dance* that Joyce (1980) suggested gives each student a chance to receive attention from everyone and allows the teacher the opportunity to give each student a moment of undivided attention.

Relaxation *(about 5 minutes)* - Some type of quiet time should be provided to end the lesson. The purpose of a relaxation period is to provide a time to calm down following the peak of the lesson. Relaxation activities provide the closing of one activity and the preparation for a new activity which will follow. Relaxation activities not only provide a calming influence, but refresh the body and the mind. Another term such as "cool-down" or "quiet time" can be used for the relaxation period. The teacher can also use a phrase such as "the special quiet moment" or tell the students to find their "quiet position." The students may suggest a term or phrase that indicates a relaxation experience.

Do not allow the students to talk or laugh during the relaxation time; rather, encourage concentration and the seeking of a quiet inner self during this activity. Specific relaxation activities are suggested at the end of several of the sample lessons and also in Chapter 10. Teachers can also create their own relaxation activities.

Evaluation of the Lesson - An evaluation section at the bottom of the lesson plan format provides a space for the teacher to reflect on the lesson. Evaluation needs to be conducted in a positive way; therefore, two questions are posed on the lesson plan form to guide the teacher in evaluating the success of the lesson:

1. What went well?

2. What can be improved?

When the lesson has been taught, teachers can answer the two questions that appear in the space at the end of the lesson. What parts of the lesson went well? What parts of the lesson could be improved? Teachers can think in terms of the: preparations and organization used to plan the lesson, time (for each section and the whole lesson), activities presented (too many, too few, just right), response of the students, teacher's response to the lesson, total lesson content, most successful part(s), which parts of the lesson are "keepers," and ideas for new lessons.

A Lesson Plan - A lesson plan is created for one period of time such as the suggested 25 to 30 minute lessons in this book, and is usually part of a **Unit.** A Unit plan consists of several individual lessons that are designed to lead to some type of conclusion or culmination.

Four units are presented in this book (Body, Time, Space, and Force) with two sample lessons for each unit. Hopefully, teachers will add to these units by creating their own lessons, as well as creating other units and lessons concerning topics about which to dance. Units can cover any topic: language arts, mathematics, music, art, science, current events, weather, seasons, holidays, and many other subjects. The lessons in the appendix which were created by some Idaho Classroom Teachers will help provide topical ideas for units as well as offer examples of tried and tested lessons.

Although the four activities of the lesson model have been described separately, the teacher should recognize that they are integral parts of a single lesson. The following illustration provides a visual image of the activities of the lesson in terms of the amount of time spent and the intensity of the activity.

Illustration of the Visual Image of the Lesson Activities

		GATHERING ACTIVITY Beginning Middle Ending	
WARM-UPS	MOVEMENT EXPLORATION	Show and Share	RELAXATION
5 Minutes	5-7 Minutes	10-15 Minutes	5 Minutes
Part 1	Part 2	Part 3	Part 4

Note that the warm-ups in the lesson begin gently and build into the movement exploration activities. Based on the exploration phase, students gather together movement sequences that contain a beginning, a middle, and an ending; and these come together in the gathering activity. Students then perform for other class members the movement patterns that they have created. Relaxation activities complete the lesson.

The proportion of time allotted to each lesson part (as shown in the illustration) is an approximation. According to this plan, the largest portion of time is spent in the gathering activity phase of the lesson. Teachers should try this time allotment for the first few lessons and later adjust the minutes based upon their style of teaching, the time available, and the needs and skill level of the students.

An outline of the lesson plan format is provided at the end of the chapter for further study and use. The form is designed to assist the teacher in briefly writing down the plans for each part of the creative movement activity. This form is used throughout the book, with a handwritten sample outline following each detailed lesson in Chapters 4 through 7.

On the form, space is provided at the beginning for the unit title, the lesson title, the date of the lesson, and the objectives. While the space is limited to approximately three or four objectives, if more objectives are planned the teacher can "sandwich in" information. The date is important in order to keep track of when and to whom each lesson is taught. New ideas stem from "reteaching" any lessons, because each group is different each time it is taught; even when a section within a lesson is repeated, it will develop a unique flavor.

The four activity categories for each lesson—warm-ups, movement exploration activities, gathering activity, and relaxation—provide space for the teachers to write a sentence or guiding words in the space provided for each activity. A supply of blank lesson plan forms are provided at the end of the book and can remain attached in the book or be removed for the teacher to use.

Other Parts of the Lesson Plan

Also appearing on the lesson plan form is a section in the upper right-hand corner for the age group which was taught and the number of students in the class. In the "organization box" space is provided to list props/materials, visual aids, equipment, and accompaniment that will be needed for the lesson. A word or term under each heading might be sufficient, but if more space is needed the teacher could continue more detailed notes on the back of the form. A few examples of props, visual aids, equipment, and accompaniment follow:

> **Props/Materials** could include scarves, streamers, hoops, or other items needed for the teacher and/or the students.
>
> **Visual aids** could include charts, posters, diagrams on the chalkboard, pictures, slides to be projected, or other visual media needed for the lesson.
>
> **Equipment** could include record, cassette, or CD players , slide projectors, percussion instruments, specific records or cassette tapes, or CDs, and video players, cameras, and monitors.
>
> *(continued)*

> **Accompaniment** could include music, percussion instruments, clapping, using the voice, or other methods that will be discussed in the sample lessons.
>
> [Accompaniment is discussed more extensively later in this chapter and props and visual aids are addressed in Chapter 8.]

A place for formation and time also appears on the lesson plan format. **Formation** refers to how the students are arranged, such as sitting or standing in a circle, in pairs, small groups, lines, or scattered throughout the room. **Time** refers to the estimated number of minutes that are planned for each part of the lesson.

Remember that the time for lessons can be adjusted by the teacher as necessary. Providing creative dance activities each day for a few minutes is better than no dancing at all. Some teachers have expressed concern that they simply do not have a block of 30 minutes to teach creative dance. My advice is to "grab" as much time as you can and later expand the dance activities as much as possible. Always have a brief warm up and relaxation time, however, no matter what other activities are chosen. Building on "yesterday's" experience is important; consequently, teaching one part of the lesson today and another part tomorrow may be the choice that will work best. Just keep dancing!

This lesson plan format has proven to be very successful for helping teachers prepare creative movement lessons. Teachers are encouraged, however, to use the format that works best for them and are welcome to modify this form as needed.

SPACE FOR CREATIVE MOVEMENT

The teacher should try to create an open space for the movement activity. Chairs and tables may need to be moved to the edge of the room leaving a center area in which to teach. The ideal space for movement activities is a large room, a gymnasium, or an outdoor play area, with as few obstructions as possible. Beware of a space that is too large, though, because it can become overwhelming. Any space, however, can be used within its limits. The type of space available may even influence lesson content and other procedures. For example, if an outdoor play area is used, asking the students to sit down or lie on the ground may not be appropriate if the surface is dusty or dirty. Some classroom settings also can be limiting, but they may provide opportunities for innovative movement activities by using tables and chairs as props for expressing such terms as "over," "under," "around," "behind," "between," or "through."

The teacher needs to become aware of the useful space in the area where the activity will take place. As the creative movement experiences develop, both the teacher and the students will discover creative ways to use the available space.

Always check the floor or movement surface for safety hazards before the lesson begins. Thumb tacks, staples, pins, or other potentially dangerous items can fall on the floor without notice. Make sure that protruding objects or holes in the ground or playground area, that might interfere with the students moving in the space available, are avoided. A slippery floor can also cause accidents, so care must be taken when deciding whether to have the students keep their socks and shoes on or remove them for the movement activities. Socks, however, should not be allowed on highly polished floors such as tile or gymnasium floors.

The teacher should help students recognize any equipment or furnishings in the room or space that could be hazardous and show the students all of the places that they can use for movement, and all of the places where they should not go.

TEACHING CUES

Before beginning the first lesson in creative movement, the teacher needs to set the ground rules with the students. Students need to know where to go and where not to go, how to start and stop, how to make formations, how to prepare their feet for movement, and any other rules for safe conduct.

Where to Go and Where Not to Go

A follow-the-teacher (leader) activity can be used to show younger students where they may go and where they may not go. March music is a suitable accompaniment. The students can line up behind the teacher who takes them around the space showing them where they can go and places that are "off limits." With all ages of students, the main point to clarify is the limits of the space to be used for the movement activity.

How to Start and Stop

Getting-started cues are important and provide the necessary structure for having a good beginning. The following cues are suggested phrases for a teacher to say to the students: "Ready? Begin." "When I count to three (or some other number the teacher may select) you will begin, 1-2-3." "When the drum or music begins, you may start."

Learning how to stop is an equally important part of every movement activity. Cues such as "when the music stops," or "when the drum stops, you stop," or "freeze when you hear one very loud beat on the drum," or "keep moving until I count to five (or whatever number the teacher selects) and then stop."

The teacher may need to help younger students explore the term "freeze" by asking a question like "What can you think of that is frozen?" (Some answers could be ice cubes, ice cream, or frozen foods. On television a "freeze frame" may appear to show the viewers some action that is better seen when it is stopped.) "How does something frozen move?" (It doesn't!) A practice session is one way to implement learning how to stop. The students may also think of cues for stopping.

The skills of listening for cues and following directions are being learned all of the time that the students are involved in movement activities. Cues must be established and used consistently, however, in order to solicit the desired response from the students and to avoid confusion. If the students have difficulty following directions or seem out of control, the teacher should always have everyone "Stop" or "Freeze," sit down if necessary, and explain the directions and try the activity again.

Formations

Circles, lines, pairs, groups, or scattered formations can be used during the creative movement experiences. The best formation to use when starting a lesson is to have the students sitting in a **circle.** Ending a creative movement lesson with the students in a circle also works well.

For a **scattered** formation students may select their own places in the room. Pieces of masking tape (or colored stickers or labels) placed on the floor throughout the room can be used to help younger students find a separate spot of their own (as opposed to clinging together in a group). As a cue for changing from a circle to a scattered formation, the teacher can say:

> **When I count three, I want everyone to tip-toe (or some other locomotor movement) to a spot you see. Stop and sit on that spot while making an interesting shape. Only one person can be on a spot. Ready, 1-2-3, tip-toe to your spot.**

If a **line** formation is required, long pieces of masking tape can be used to designate the lines, and the students can be instructed to move to those lines in whatever way the teacher chooses. If a natural line such as a joint or a crack is already on the classroom floor, the teacher can use it for the formation.

Preparing the Feet for Movement

Preferably students should participate in creative movement activities in bare feet, and procedures for removing shoes and socks should be established. If the surface is slippery or rough, however, the students should keep their shoes on. Do not allow students to participate in creative movement activities wearing socks unless the movement space is carpeted. When the shoes and socks have been removed and placed outside of the designated movement area, the students can enter the movement space and sit down in a circle to show that they are ready.

When the lesson is over, the students may be given a movement task to take them to their shoes. Such tasks as asking all of the girls to skip to their shoes, or telling the boys to hop to their shoes, keep the students busy and interested in one last movement activity. Also many innovative movement tasks for putting on shoes can be created by the teacher and the students. The teacher may need to allow time to assist some of the younger students, however, with taking off and putting on shoes.

The important idea is to use cues that seem appropriate for the teacher and the age group of the class. As soon as the starting, stopping, and listening cues are learned, the teacher will always be able to properly lead and control the students during the movement experiences.

Rules for Students

Sullivan (1982) recommended the following list of rules for students participating in movement experiences.

Children should not wear or carry dangerous items.

Children must not be allowed to deliberately hurt one another physically.

Children must not be allowed to tease or ridicule one another.

Children must come where the teacher is upon hearing a prearranged signal or when the teacher asks them to.

Children are expected to behave with an appropriate degree of commitment to the activities.

Older children must obey the direction "Freeze!" (p. 9)

No student should be allowed to disturb others during the creative movement activities. Each student is expected to learn about managing his or her own body and space and to allow the other students to take care of themselves. The teacher will want to work to preserve all of these rules, which will help insure safe and successful movement experiences for everyone.

The teacher should expect every student to participate, and students should not be punished by being removed from the activity if this procedure can be avoided. If students choose not to participate, however, they should not be forced into the experience. The goal is to entice the shy student by the joy and fun that everyone else is having with creative movement. Eventually all students will want to join the activity.

NOTES FOR THE TEACHER

1. Keep the lesson simple and state objectives clearly.

2. Allow the students sufficient time to fully explore the selected movement.

3. Keep the directions brief and simple to allow more time for movement with less talking.

4. Evaluate the lesson afterwards.

Joyce (1980) suggested that at the end of each lesson, teachers ask themselves the following questions as a way to evaluate achievement:

Did we fully explore an element? [movement-of-the-day selected by the teacher]

Did they try movements they would not have tried without my questions?

Did I challenge them to extend their ability?

Did they select and use movements of their own choice at some point during the lesson? (p. 39)

Teachers should remember that they act as guides in creative movement by suggesting ways for students to move and then allowing them to create a pattern. Creative movement experiences are success-oriented because there is no wrong way to move. The teacher should frequently use positive reinforcements by telling the students, "I like the way that Lisa is moving," or "Look at the interesting shape that Arthur has made." This acceptance helps the students develop self-confidence and pride in their skills.

ACCOMPANIMENT FOR CREATIVE MOVEMENT ACTIVITIES

Many types of accompaniment can be used for creative movement activities. Music may be the first type of accompaniment that comes to mind. Music on compact discs (CDs), records, and cassette tapes is readily available. Classical composers such as Debussy, Chopin, Beethoven, Bach, Grieg, Vivaldi, Mozart, Tchaikovsky, and others have created music that can be used for any part of the lesson, from warm ups to relaxation.

In Chapter 7, Lesson One—Force Through Movement, "In the Hall of the Mountain King" Op. 46/4 from the Peer Gynt Suite by Edvard Grieg was selected as accompaniment for exploring strong, forceful, (percussive) movements. In contrast to Grieg's percussive music, the "Pachelbel Canon" is an excellent accompaniment for sustained movement, mirroring with partners, or relaxation activities.

Music selections from ballets such as "Swan Lake," "Giselle," "The Nutcracker," or others could provide accompaniment for any part of the lesson. The overture at the beginning of classical music selections provides a sampling of the music to be heard in its entirety. If possible, the teacher should ask to listen to selections on CDs, records, or tapes before purchasing, and make a decision concerning whether or not the music seems appropriate for the lesson(s) planned.

Popular music is another source of accompaniment. Usually music without lyrics is more suitable; however, some selections with words may be appropriate. For example, "Morning," by Al Jarreau has been used successfully for warm-up activities. Music by percussionist Andreas Vollenweider provides excellent accompaniment; harps, gamelans, bells, wind chimes, and many other instruments offer an exciting musical background for creating movement. Some of the Vollenweider albums include "Down to the Moon," "White Winds," and "Behind the Garden Wall" and are available in the world market. Paul Hardcastle has composed good instrumental music for movement activities. One album, titled "Rainforest," provides a fine selection of pieces containing a strong, steady beat. Another composer, Ray Lynch, has created excellent music which can serve as accompaniment for a variety of movement activities; his albums include "The Sky of Mind," "Deep Breakfast," and "No Blue Thing."

Some recent (in 1995) "finds" in music for this author are "Contrast & Continuum, Volume I and Volume II, Music for Creative Dance," composed and marketed by Eric Chappelle. Each volume includes a booklet on suggested movements. See the appendix for ordering these albums on cassette or CD. Composer Kurt Bestor has marvelous lyrical music written for dancing as well as listening. He has several albums available including "Seasons" that focuses on Spring, Summer, Autumn, and Winter.

Traditional music from any culture can also provide wonderful accompaniment for creative movement activities. Many of these traditional music pieces have a good steady beat that can accompany various lesson parts, as well as acquaint students with music from other cultures. The author's collection of cultural music includes selections from Malaysia, Cambodia, Bali, Thailand, China, Greece, Turkey, Scotland, England, Mexico, and Bolivia. Look for unique music when traveling within or outside of the United States.

Finally, some music has also been especially developed and produced for creative movement and creative dance activities. Teachers can obtain catalogues and price lists from the record and music companies listed in the resources section. Also, music for children's songs, games, and dances is available in the music sections of most department stores.

One of the best sources of suggested musical accompaniment is Gilbert's (1992) book, *Creative Dance for All Ages*, Appendix F—Instrumental and Activity Music List. She has listed musical selections for a variety of concepts such as place, size, level, direction, pathways, focus, speed, rhythm, energy, weight, flow, body parts, body shapes, balance, relationships, locomotor/nonlocomotor, free dance, instruments, rest/alignment, and pause.

Other Types of Accompaniment

In addition to singing, vocal accompaniment also includes counting, poetry, and chanting by the teacher and/or the students.

Percussion accompaniment includes drums, rhythm instruments, clapping, or anything that produces a sound when it is struck. Students can make a variety of percussion instruments with sticks, rattles made by filling plastic containers or cans with rice or beans, and drums created from plastic containers or cans and wooden spoons as the drumsticks.

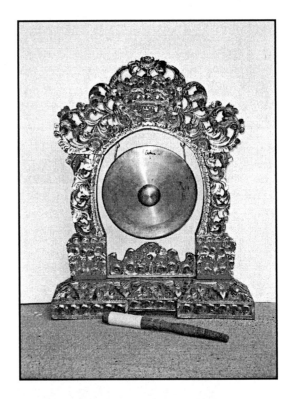

Balinese Gong

A Balinese gong made from "scratch" by hand and purchased by the author in Bali from a family-owned company. This gong is a "home made instrument" in the finest sense.

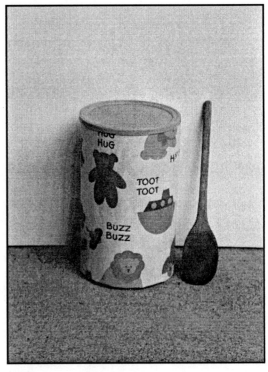

A Drum

A drink container or an oatmeal box with the lid on the top becomes a drum. This "drum" is covered with gift wrapping paper. A wooden spoon is the beater.

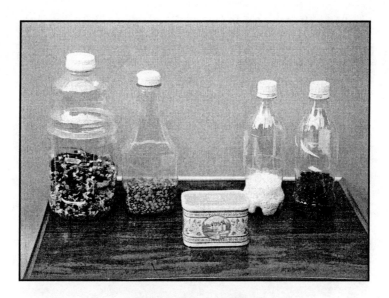

Shakers or Rattles
Use plastic or metal containers which are filled with beans, rice, or peas. The neck of the bottles make a good grip for the musician.

Graham, Holt/Hale, and Parker (1993) suggested easy-to-make rhythm instruments that include:

Pie pan shaker—Place small round stones or dried beans in an aluminum pie pan, [cover with another pie pan and staple closed].

Balloon shaker—pour sand, rice, beans . . . into a balloon. Partially inflate the balloon and tie the end.

Bleach (or milk) jug drum—Screw top of jug and secure with tape or glue. Hit with a dowel rod. Children can decorate the jug with paint or colored tape (p. 479).

Fleming (1976) provides a wealth of information through her illustrations and easy-to-follow directions for making a wide variety percussion instruments including drums, rattles, shakers, rhythm sticks, cymbals, and stringed instruments (pp. 246- 263). Many ideas are presented that could be excellent class projects for the students to recycle materials that would be involved in making instruments as a part of creative movement experiences.

Silence is also an accompaniment. Silence can be used to allow students to concentrate on creating or performing certain movement patterns without interruption.

The selecting of accompaniment should be enjoyable and interesting for teachers and students. Students will have many ideas to contribute to the selection of the accompaniment.

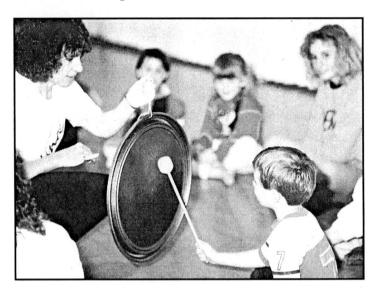

Using a Gong

The "gong" is a large lid that came from a flour container. A hole was drilled and a cord atached to suspend the instrument.

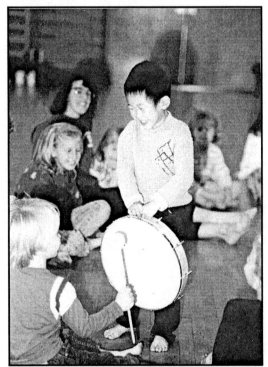

Using a Drum

SUMMARY

This chapter presented a lesson format for developing creative movement activities. Creative experiences must be carefully planned. The lesson format that has been introduced provides such a structure. A lesson should include (a) a warm up, (b) an exploration of the movement topic-of-the-day (and time for the students to explore all of its possibilities), (c) a gathering activity in which the student puts movement into form by developing a beginning, a middle, and an ending (shape-movement-shape), with some time provided for sharing the movement pieces with the class, and (d) relaxation activities to end each lesson. The illustration provided in this chapter shows the time for each part of the lesson and how the lesson builds to a peak and closes with relaxation activities.

Ideally, creative movement should take place in an area that permits freedom of movement in a safe environment. The teacher should acquaint the students with where to move and where not to move. Teaching cues to help the students start, stop, listen, and change formations were suggested.

When preparing a lesson in creative movement, teachers should keep every aspect of the lesson as simple and direct as possible. Teachers are guides and should accept the movement responses of the students. Positive reinforcement should be given to the students to instill self confidence.

Also discussed were ideas for various types of accompaniment for creative movement activities, such as classical, popular, and cultural music; percussion instruments; speaking; or silence.

An outline of the lesson plan format was presented as a suggestion to the teacher. Teachers should feel free to adapt the lesson plan format to fit their teaching styles.

CREATIVE DANCE - LESSON PLAN OUTLINE

Unit title: *Lesson title:* *Date:*	*Props/Materials:* *Visual Aids:*
Objectives	*Equipment:* *Accompaniment:*

Activities of the Lesson	Formation	Time
WARM-UPS		
MOVEMENT EXPLORATION ACTIVITIES		
GATHERING ACTIVITY		
RELAXATION		
Evaluation of the lesson: 1. What went well? 2. What can be improved?		

Chapter 4

THE BODY

INTRODUCTION

The body is the instrument used in creative movement to express ideas, thoughts, and feelings. This chapter includes two sample lessons focusing on the element of the body: (1) My Body Moves and (2) Copycat.

The sample lessons are presented in detail with examples of what the teacher can say to the students. In fact, each lesson is written in a form that can be used almost word-for-word. The sample lessons are also designed as models for teachers to use in developing further lessons, and they can be adapted to any teaching style, age group, and ability. Consequently, the teacher should feel free to be innovative in planning and implementing creative movement activities as soon as the sample lessons have been taught.

The lessons in this book proceed sequentially by building from a single-movement concept to a combination of movements. Therefore, the teacher will be able to begin with a very simple activity and progress to greater complexity as the students are ready. Chapters 4 through 7 address the individual elements of creative movement—body, time, space, and force. Although each chapter attempts to focus attention on just one element, these elements overlap and cannot be separated completely.

Following each lesson, a detailed outline of the lesson is written on the Lesson Plan Form as an example of how the teacher might write a lesson. (Additional sample lessons designed by teachers appear in an appendix.) Although these outlines can be used exactly as they are presented, they may also serve as models for teachers to prepare additional, more unique lessons for themselves. Also, extra copies of the lesson plan form are located in an appendix at the end of the book.

All of the detailed lessons and outlines are meant to be extended, adapted for any age group and ability, or become "spin-offs" for other lessons by the teacher as experience and confidence in teaching creative movement activities are gained. As the teacher becomes independent of the sample lessons, the movement activities will flow more easily and will become the teacher's personal property.

Other ideas for movement that focus on the body, body parts, body actions, or body shapes are included in a later section of this chapter "Body Words for Movement Exploration." Each word in that section can be used as a foundation for creating further creative movement lessons for the body element.

"The Idea Pages," at the end of Chapters 4 through 11, are also provided for the teacher to record ideas for lesson content as they are discovered during the reading of the chapter or as the sample lessons in the chapter are taught. The ideas will come both from the teacher and the students. Do not be surprised if you run out of space on The Idea Pages.

Remember that the number of minutes suggested for each section of the lesson is an estimate. The sensitivity of the teacher to the activity of the students will indicate when to move to the next part of the lesson. This skill will develop as more creative movement activities are presented. If the students are engrossed in a particular part of a lesson, allow them to remain there for the time needed to complete the experience.

The lesson plans are only guidelines that can be changed in any way on a moment's notice. This is part of being a **creative teacher.** The only parts of the lesson plan that should remain intact are the brief warm up at the beginning and the relaxation period at the end of the lesson. The relaxation period brings physical, mental, and emotional fulfillment to the activity and closure for both the teacher and the students.

The lesson format used in this book includes:

1. Warm-Ups

2. Movement Exploration Activities

3. Gathering Activity (a culminating experience)

4. Relaxation

Following the completion of each lesson, the teacher should briefly evaluate the success of the lesson by recording what went well and what can be improved to make a better lesson the next time it is taught. Since the lessons assume that the teacher will move among the students during instruction when appropriate, the evaluation will be based on the observations made by the teacher as to how successful the lesson was with his or her group of students.

LESSON ONE — MY BODY MOVES

OBJECTIVES

1. To identify body parts
2. To explore different ways of moving body parts
3. To explore shapes and levels
4. To create a simple movement sequence using nonlocomotor and locomotor movements combined with shapes and levels

WARM-UPS *(5 Minutes)*

Three warm-up activities are being introduced with this lesson and include both nonlocomotor and locomotor activities. The teacher is encouraged to try all three of these activities. The purpose of the warm-up activity is to loosen the muscles and the mind and prepare the students for action. These warm-up activities can also be used in other lessons. A new set of warm-up activities for every lesson is not necessary, however, because students enjoy repetition of movement activities.

ACTIVITY 1 (Identify body parts, stretching and bending body and parts)

Accompaniment: Voices and Music
Directions:

Part 1. (Sitting in a circle with legs stretched forward) Have the students follow your actions of touching specific body parts while you say the following words using a rhythmic chant of your voice. You may also sing the words to the the tune of "London Bridge is Falling Down."

> **Head and shoulders, knees and toes,**
> **knees and toes, knees and toes;**
> **Head and shoulders, knees and toes,**
> **clap your hands together.**

Repeat this chant again.

Now with legs crossed, have the students follow your actions as you chant the second part of the activity as follows:

Eyes and ears, and nose and chin,
nose and chin, nose and chin;
Eyes and ears, and nose and chin;
Now show me a great big grin.
(or if the floor surface allows children to spin on their seats,
you can say)
Now show me a great big spin.

Repeat the second part of the chant again. Then repeat both parts of the chant beginning with the head. This activity can be performed sitting and/or standing depending upon the conditions of the space, time available, or the preference of the students or teacher.

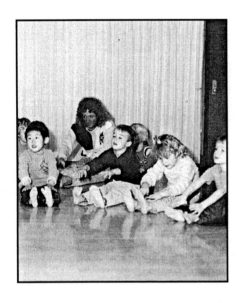

**Head and Shoulders,
Knees and Toes**

**Eyes and Ears,
Nose and Chin**

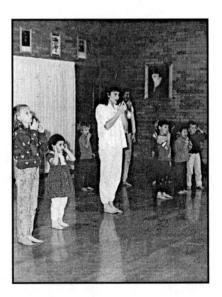

Part 2. (Standing in a circle with feet about shoulder width apart, knees relaxed) This activity includes four parts (or measures of beats) using 8 counts and 4 counts. The pattern is:

> **8 counts of stretching** arms above the head
> **4 counts bending** knees and elbows
> **4 counts to "hang over" and shake** heads and arms, and
> **8 counts to uncurl** slowly returning to a standing position.

8 counts of stretching—Standing and reaching both arms up to the ceiling , have the students stretch the right arm, then the left arm, and alternate arms for each count until the teacher has counted to eight (students can count too, if desired). The sequence can be accompanied by the teacher counting and/or giving verbal cues; music with a good steady beat (not too fast) could provide accompaniment. The teacher may say:

Ready? Stretch 1, 2, 3, 4, 5, 6, 7, 8

(Finish, as the exercise began, with both arms reaching toward the ceiling.)

[**Note:** Right and left directions may mean very little to preschool students, but the teacher can encourage young students to alternate the use of body parts. For the sake of the teachers however, directions for the lessons are given as right and left.]

4 counts bending—Standing with arms reaching overhead, have the students use four counts to bend elbows and knees simulateously. The body will be lowered a little bit as the knees bend. The teacher may say:

Bend elbows and knees 2-3-4

4 counts to "hang over" and shake—Keeping the knees bent, have the students curl down by dropping their chins toward their chests, caving in their stomachs and allowing their arms to carefully drop to the floor. The backs of fingers or hands are resting on the floor, with arms feeling heavy and shoulders relaxed, knees are bent, back is curved, top of the head is toward the floor and shake heads and arms. The teacher may say:

Hang and shake 2-3-4

8 counts to uncurl—Have students slowly begin straightening knees as they begin to return to a standing position. As the knees straighten, the base of the spine begins to straighten as students continue uncurling. Have the students keep their heads down and arms relaxed and heavy as they uncurl. The last body parts to uncurl will be the neck (about count 7) and the head (on count 8). The teacher may say:

Uncurl slowly (straighten knees) 2-3-4, (back) 5-6, (neck) 7, (head) 8

Repeat the entire activity again using the cues of the 8 counts for stretching, 4 counts for bending, 4 counts for hanging and shaking, and 8 counts for uncurling.

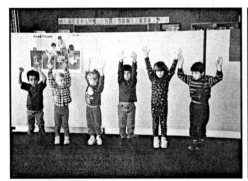

**Part 1
8 counts to stretch 8 times**

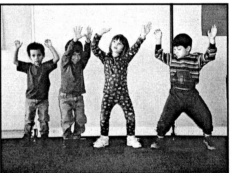

**Part 2
4 counts to bend elbows
and knees**

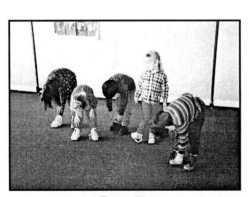

**Part 3
4 counts to
"hang over" and shake**

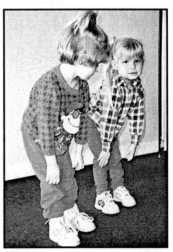

**Part 4
8 counts to uncurl slowly**

ACTIVITY 2 "Twist, Snap, Stamp, and Clap" (Twisting and turning body parts)

Accompaniment: Music, voice, clapping or percussion instruments such as a drum or sticks

Directions: (Standing in a circle with arms extended away from sides; arms parallel to the floor) The teacher can demonstrate the activities and tell the students the following:

Keep your feet firmly planted on the floor and twist your body slowly to the right side; twist to the left side; now turn around in place to your right, taking 4 small steps in a circle. Here is a chant we can use for the accompaniment:

twist,	twist,	turn-a-round
(right)	(left)	(to the right)
1 - 2	3 - 4	5 - 6 - 7 - 8
twist,	twist,	turn-a-round
(left)	(right)	(to the left)
1 - 2	3 - 4	5 - 6 - 7 - 8

Repeat the above pattern again until the students are able to follow the teacher's cues with the proper rhythm.

Now add a snap of your fingers after you twist to the right and twist to the left, and stamp four times while turning around. The pattern now becomes:

twist-snap,	twist-snap,	stamp, stamp, stamp, stamp
(right)	(left)	(while turning right)
1 - 2	3 - 4	5 - 6 - 7 - 8
twist-snap,	twist-snap,	stamp, stamp, stamp, stamp
(left)	(right)	(while turning left)
1 - 2	3 - 4	5 - 6 - 7 - 8

Repeat the twist-and-snap finger pattern again until the students are able to follow the teacher's cues. An additional challenge is created for the third part of this pattern by adding four claps of the hands simultaneously with the stamps in a circle (one clap with each stamp). Begin to the right, then to the left; repeat right and left. The pattern is:

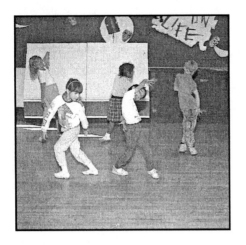

Twisting

twist-snap, (right)	twist-snap, (left)	stamp, stamp, stamp, stamp clap, clap, clap, clap (while turning right)
1 - 2	3 - 4	5 - 6 - 7 - 8
twist-snap, (left)	twist-snap (right)	stamp, stamp, stamp, stamp clap, clap, clap, clap (while turning left)
1 - 2	3 - 4	5 - 6 - 7 - 8

Again, repeat the pattern until the students are able to follow the cues.

Combine one set of each pattern (right and left) with finger snaps and hand claps. This pattern will now have a total of six measures (or 6 units of 8 beats each) in the sequence: two measures for the twist pattern (one measure right; one measure left); two measures for the twist-snap-stamp combination; and two measures for the twist-snap-stamp-clap combination.

ACTIVITY 3 (Walking without touching anyone or anything)

Accompaniment: Poetry reading, drum or music with a clear, steady beat
Directions:

Part 1. (Scattered and seated for poetry reading) The teacher can begin the lesson by saying:

> **Today I will read a poem to you while you listen. Then we will experiment with different movements. The poem is "Do Not Bump."**
>
> > **The game is not to bump another,**
> > **Never touch or crowd the other.**
> >
> > **This may be quite hard, I know,**
> > **But eyes will tell you where to go.**
> > **Use your eyes and find a space;**
> > **With hand outstretched to lead the way,**
> > **Tiptoe quickly there to stay,**
> > **But Never, Never BUMP!**
>
> *by permission of Grace C. Nash, author.*
> *From Verses and Movement, Grace Nash Publications,*
> *Scottsdale, Arizona 85252, U.S.A.*

Nash (1972) suggested the following ideas for ways to use movement with her poem:

> Use one third of the class in the beginning to allow sufficient space in which to move. After success in their first tries, the numbers can gradually be increased until all of the children can move [simultaneously] without touching each other . . . an important skill and one which aids in the development of control and freedom in movement.
>
> The next step is the use of different kinds of movement in going to and returning from a new place in the room. Experiment in contrasts of walking for example; (a) heavy exhausting steps going; delicate, light steps returning; (b) a twisted route, straight route; (c) fast walk, slow walk. Try combinations of these as children gain in skill (p. 10).

Note: Other movement poems can be used in place of the one suggested, or the teacher can omit the poetry section of this lesson and begin with the next section listed below.

Part 2. The teacher can now have the students stand and prepare them for the next instructions:

> **When I say "Go," everyone will begin walking forward around the room without touching anyone or anything.** (The teacher can specify clockwise or counterclockwise.) **When the drum (or music) stops, you will stop and "freeze." What does freeze mean?** (Discuss this concept with the students.) **How many of you think you can do this? Good. Ready? Go.**

Part 3. Allow the students to walk for a while, then have them "freeze" for the next instruction.

> **When I say "Go," begin walking anywhere in our movement space that you wish. When I say "freeze" you will stop and make a shape with your body. Ready? Go.** (Allow the students a few seconds for the first attempt. You can extend the time as they show that they can avoid bumping.) **Freeze! Good.**

The teacher can beat a drum or clap his or her hands to give the students a rhythm to follow.

Part 4. For the next part of the activity, instruct the students as follows:

> **Can you walk backwards without bumping into anyone? Let us try. Ready? Go.** (Allow the students to walk backwards as the teacher provides a drum beat or clapping rhythm.) **Freeze and make a shape. Good, Look at all of the interesting shapes! Do you think that you can walk forward, then backward, then freeze and make a shape? I will tell you when to walk forward, backward, freeze and make a shape. Ready? Walk forward.** (Allow the students to move around the room before having them change directions.) **Now walk backwards without bumping into anyone. Freeze and make a shape.**

Repeat this pattern a few times and vary the order of the movements and the length of time that each part is performed.

Part 5. Finish the exercise with the following instruction:

> **When I count three, walk to the circle and sit down in your own space without touching anyone. Ready? One-two-three.**

MOVEMENT EXPLORATION ACTIVITIES
(5-7 Minutes)

Part 1. (Sitting) Show pictures of people; and as you point to the body parts in the pictures, ask the students to point to their own body parts:

> **Point to your head, eyes, ears, nose, chin, neck, shoulders, upper arms, elbows, lower arms, wrists, fingers, chest, stomach, hips, upper legs (thighs), knees, lower legs, ankles, feet, toes.**

This is a very important activity for younger students. Teachers of older students may only need to spend a short time identifying body parts and can extend this exploration by teaching information about various bones and muscles.

A variety of anatomy charts are available with notations naming the bones and muscles. Charts are available for children through adults illustrating simple to complex concepts. The teacher and students could point to bones in the arm such as the humerus, radius, and ulna; bones in the leg such as the femur, tibia, and fibula. Muscles like the trapezius, biceps, or gastrocnemius (calf) could be located. An activity could be created to the spiritual song of "The head bone's connected to the neck bone."

Part 2. (Sitting) Begin exploring movements of different body parts by asking questions such as:

> **How many different ways can your** (name whatever body part you want) **move? Forward? Backward? To the Side? In a Circle? Up and down? Back and forth?** (Suggestion: begin with the head and work down.)

Further questions to ask students about the body are listed at the end of this chapter. These questions will assist the teacher in more fully developing this movement exploration activity.

Part 3. (Sitting) Each time the drum beats (or hands clap), ask the students to bend, stretch, or twist a body part. For example, the teacher can say "bend," or "stretch," or "twist," and allow the students to select the body part, or the teacher can select the body part and allow the students to choose bend, stretch, or twist. Explore as many possibilities as time and interest permit.

Part 4. (Standing) Repeat activity three in a standing position. The teacher can ask students questions, such as:

Can you bend one body part?
Can you bend an upper body part and a lower body part?
Can you bend one body part and stretch another body part?
Can you show me a twisted body shape?

Next, continue exploring body shapes by combining the shapes with the different levels at which the body can move—high, medium, and low. The teacher can challenge the students by making statements such as:

Show me a low twisted shape
Try a high stretched shape.
Let me see a bent shape at a medium level.

The teacher and students can develop many combinations through experimentation.

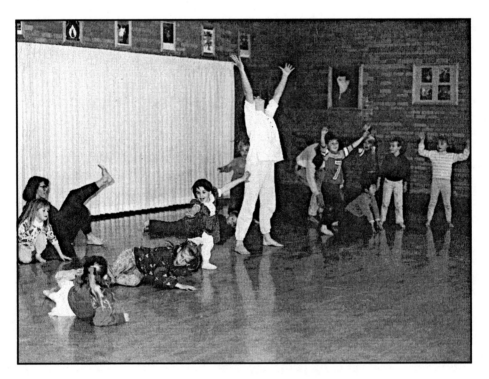

Levels and Shapes

Part 5. (Standing) Allow the students to explore a locomotor movement. Begin with walking. Walk forward, then backward. (In later lessons, other pathways of movement can be explored, such as moving sideways, in a small circle, in a curving, straight, or angular pathway.) Music or a drum beat can be used as accompaniment. Encourage the students to move through the available space without touching or bumping anyone. When the music or drum beat stops, the students should "freeze" until the next direction is given and they are told "ready, begin." In later lessons, other locomotor movements such as running, leaping, hopping, jumping, skipping, sliding, or galloping (or a combination of two or three of these movements) will be incorporated.

GATHERING ACTIVITY *(10-15 Minutes)*

Finish the lesson by gathering together the parts of the lesson that were presented independently and putting them together into a form. From the movement that the students have already developed, create a movement sequence that includes a beginning, a middle, and an ending.

CREATING A MOVEMENT PATTERN

Ask the students to walk to a new place in the room, and then stop. **"Show me a low stretched shape"** (or another level and shape the teacher suggests—the combinations are numerous). This low stretched shape is the *beginning*. **"When the drum beats you will be walk to another place in the room." "Ready? Go."** This walking movement is the *middle* portion of the movement pattern. **"When the drum stops, show me a high twisted shape."** This is the *ending* of the pattern.

Shape-movement-shape is the basic sequence for any movement pattern. The pattern described above can be summarized in the following way:

Beginning shape:	low, stretched
Movement:	walk forward
Ending shape:	high, twisted

The shape-movement-shape sequence is a simple, clear way to begin creating movement patterns. The combinations of locomotor movements, body shapes, and levels are numerous. These combinations can be created by the teacher, the students, or preferably both.

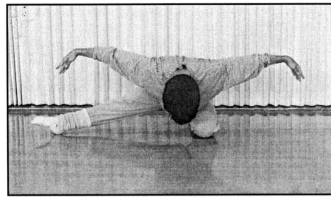

Low Stretched Shape

Combination of High Twisted and Low Stretched Shape

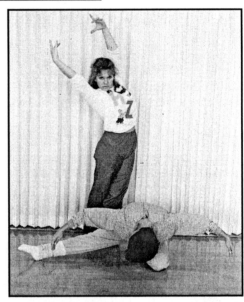

Extended pattern - Any movement sequence can be extended in a variety of ways to add interest and challenge to the creative development of the students. The pattern just described contains the basic shape-movement-shape concept but is now being extended by adding one more shape and one more locomotor movement. Accompaniment can be provided by the teacher counting, beating a drum, clapping, or using carefully selected music. The extended pattern (or the 3-shape pattern) is:

Beginning
Shape 1—**Make a low stretched shape, hold for 4 counts.**
Movement—**Walk forward in any direction for 8 counts.**

Middle
Shape 2—**Make a high twisted shape, hold for 4 counts.**
Movement—**Walk backward in any direction for 8 counts.**

Ending
Shape 3—**Make a shape of your choice, hold 8 counts.**

Repeat this pattern from the beginning, and the students can use the same shape for each section or select a new shape. The teacher can change the shapes, levels, direction, locomotor movements, and the counts used for each part. Eventually the students should be allowed to assist in developing the movement patterns, and finally to create their own individual sequences of movement based on the concept of shape-movement-shape. The teacher should continually give positive reinforcement to the students regarding the interesting shapes they have created, their ability to move skillfully in the space, and their skill in creating fascinating movement sequences.

The basic and extended movement patterns are intended for students to explore individually. During the first few creative movement experiences, the goal is to individualize the activities to allow each student to take responsibility for himself or herself as a movement skill is developed.

In later lessons, further challenges using these patterns can be offered by allowing students to create patterns in pairs or groups. Groups of three to five students seem to work successfully. The students may make shapes that relate to one another during the shape sequence, then travel together during the movement sequence to a new location. Another alternative for the movement sequence could be for students to travel away from each other and then return to each other before the next shape sequence.

The students will be able to think of many ways to solve movement problems presented by the shape-movement-shape sequence. Working with others and learning to relate movements to a partner or a group can be fun and can also develop positive social interaction.

Audience-performance - (Show and Share) Divide the class into two groups: (1) audience and (2) performers. Have the first group of performers show the audience the 3-shape-movement pattern twice. (This is the extended pattern.) The same accompaniment should be used for this part of the lesson that was used in developing the 3-shape-movement sequence. The performers will then trade places with the audience, and the pattern will be repeated twice by the new performers for the new audience. This activity offers students an opportunity to share in both audience and peformance experiences. It also allows them to see other students moving creatively.

RELAXATION ACTIVITIES (5 *Minutes*)

ACTIVITY 1 (Breathing and curling)

Directions: (Sitting in a circle with legs crossed and hands in laps) Ask the students to breathe air into the body (inhale) through their noses as they sit up straight while you count slowly to four. Next, ask the students to blow the air out of their mouths (exhale) as they curl forward, while you count slowly to four. Ask the students to make a sound (such as "ahhhhh") as they exhale. This adds fun to the relaxation.

ACTIVITY 2 (Gentle neck stretches)

Directions: (Sitting in a circle with legs crossed and hands in laps) Have the students slowly move their heads gently in a circular motion. Use the following cues:

Drop your chin down toward your chest.
Put your right ear near your right shoulder.
Look up at the ceiling.
(A"neck- check" for students as they look upward is to have them place the palm of one hand on the back of their necks and tilt the chin upward only until they feel pressure on the little finger—do NOT allow students to crunch the cervical vertebraes by dropping the head backward.)
Put your left ear near the left shoulder.
Drop your chin down toward your chest.
Now repeat slowly in the other direction.

ACTIVITY 3 (Tight and loose)

Directions: (Lying down on back with legs straight and arms at sides) Using a quiet, calm voice ask the students to lie down on their backs in their own space, not touching anyone, and close their eyes. The arms are down by the sides and the legs are stretched out with ankles together. Ask the students to inhale, hold their breaths, and tighten their whole bodies. Then have the students exhale (let all the air out) and loosen or release their muscles. Cues can be:

Hold your breath and tighten your muscles.
Let go of the air and loosen your muscles.

Repeat the tightening and loosening two more times.

ACTIVITY 4 (Stretch and relax)

Directions: (Lying down on back with legs straight and arms on the floor extended above the head) Working with stretching and relaxing individual body parts is a good technique that can quietly challenge the students. Ask the students to lie down on their backs (if they are not already in that position) and use the following cues for this activity:

> **Close your eyes and stretch your arms above your head, but keep them on the floor.**
> **Stretch your right leg as far as you can and then relax that leg.**
> **Stretch your left leg as far as you can and then relax it.**
> **Stretch both legs and then relax.**
>
> **Now, stretch your right arm as far above your head as you can and relax that arm.**
> **Stretch your left arm as far above your head as you can and relax that arm.**
> **Stretch both arms as far as you can and then relax.**
> **Stretch one arm and one leg as far as you can and then relax.**
> **Stretch the other arm and leg and relax (or go limp).**
>
> **While you are all relaxed, I am coming around to check an arm or leg to see how relaxed (or limp) you are.**

The teacher checks each student by gently lifting an arm or leg to see if the student is limp. If the body part is tense or tight, quietly ask the student to let you hold that body part while they relax or release the muscles.

The teacher may select all or any one of the four relaxation activities described above. The choice depends on the time available, but at least one relaxation activity should be used to complete each lesson. These relaxation activities can be used in other sample lessons in this book and lessons that the teacher will create later.

Relaxation activities are important. They provide a quiet closing (physically, mentally, and socially) to the creative movement lesson. This technique will help complete the lesson for the students and the teacher. The relaxation activities also offer physical and mental refreshment which serves as a good preparation for the next teaching activity following the creative movement lesson.

Two options are suggested for completing the relaxation phase of the lesson. Other options will be developed as the teacher gains experience with guiding students in creative movement experiences.

Option 1 - As soon as the teacher checks each student's state of relaxation, bring the lesson to a close by a statement such as the following:

Good, I see everyone is limp and relaxed. Lie quietly now and listen to your heart beating. (Allow about 10 to 15 seconds for this listening experience.) **Now stretch your arms and stretch your legs, and then slowly sit up and cross your legs and put your hands in your lap. Now we will have the girls stand and skip over and put on their socks and shoes. Boys, you can stand and hop over and put on your socks and shoes.** (The students should be ready for the next activity of the day.)

Option 2 - Play slow music for 30 to 60 seconds while the students are lying quietly on the floor. If the students are quiet, the music can be played longer, if desired. Gradually turn the music lower and instruct the students that when they cannot hear the music anymore they are to sit up slowly. When all of the students are sitting, have them breathe in slowly (inhale) through their noses, and blow air out of their mouths (exhale), and smile to end the creative movement activity for the day. The teacher may use a movement task (such as walking, hopping, or skipping) for the students to go to their socks and shoes.

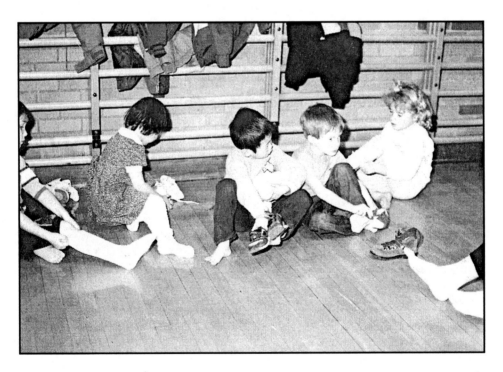

Finishing the Creative Movement Class

Outline of Lesson Plan One
"My Body Moves"

Unit title: _The Body_ **Lesson title:** _My Body Moves_ **Date:**	**Props/Materials:** **Visual Aids:** _Pictures (Poster) of people moving_
Objectives 1. _identify body parts_ 2. _explore ways of moving body parts_ 3. _explore shapes + levels_ 4. _create a movement pattern (shape-movement-shape)_	**Equipment:** _Drum, Cassette/CD Player_ **Accompaniment:** _music, voice percussion_

Activities of the Lesson	Formation	Time
WARM UPS 1. _Heads, shoulders, knees, toes_ 2. _Stretch, bend, "hang over," curl up_ 3. _Twist - snap - stamp - clap_ 4. _Walk - forward, backward, freeze_	_Circle:_ _sitting_ _standing_ _scattered_	_5 min._
MOVEMENT EXPLORATION ACTIVITIES _Show pictures - identify body parts, movements, shapes + levels_ _"How many ways can body parts move when: lying down, sitting, kneeling, standing_ _Poem "Never Bump"_ _Walk, fwd, backward - freeze in shape at high, medium, low levels_	_Sitting in a group, facing teacher._ _circle_ _scattered_	_5-7 min._

GATHERING ACTIVITY _(Shape-Movement-Shape)_
 Combination:
   SHAPE: _low - stretched_   _4 counts_
   MOVEMENT: _walk forward_   _8 counts_
   SHAPE: _high - twisted_   _4 counts_
 Add
   MOVEMENT: _walk backwards_   _8 counts_
   SHAPE: _your own_   _8 counts_
 Show + Share
	Scattered	_10-15 min._

RELAXATION _(1) Breathe, curl down + up. (2) Neck circles_ _(3) Tight + loose (4) Stretch + relax_ _(5) Slow music for 30-60 seconds_	_Circle:_ _Sitting_ _Lying on back_	_5 min._
Evaluation of the lesson: 1. What went well? 2. What can be improved?		

OBJECTIVES

1. To explore movement of body parts (swinging)
2. To explore body shapes
3. To copy the shape made by another person
4. To create a movement pattern that incorporates shapes and locomotor movements

WARM-UPS *(5 Minutes)*

Three additional warm-up activities are being introduced with this lesson. The teacher may use any one or all of these activities plus the three that were introduced with the previous lesson, My Body Moves.

ACTIVITY 1 (Swinging body parts—the arms)

Accompaniment: Music 3/4 time, or counting by the teacher
Directions: Draw a circle on the chalkboard with a horizontal line through the middle of the circle. The lower half or arc of the circle is the pathway or shape of a swinging motion. This diagram should help the students visualize the curved shape or undercurve that a swinging action takes. If the momentum from a swing is allowed to carry through, a complete circle can be made.

Part 1. (Standing in a circle with the arms hanging at the sides) Have the students swing the right arm forward while the teacher counts 1-2-3. Now have the students swing the right arm backward (1-2-3), now swing the right arm forward all the way around (1-2-3; 1-2-3). Four measures of three beats each are used for the above sequence (or a total of 12 counts). Repeat the activity using the same arm swinging backward (1-2-3), forward (1-2-3), and backward all the way around (1-2-3; 1-2-3). Repeat this pattern using the left arm swinging forward, backward, and forward all the way around; now backward, forward, and backward all the way around.

WORD CUES the teacher can use are:

FORward and BACKward and (forward) ALL the way AROUND
1-2-3   1-2-3   1-2-3   1-2-3
BACKward and FORward and (backward) ALL the way AROUND
1-2-3   1-2-3   1-2-3   1-2-3

The rhythmic accent is the bold capitalized word above. The directional words in parentheses need not be spoken.

Part 2. Beginning with the arms hanging by the sides, have the students swing both arms forward (1-2-3), backward (1-2-3), and forward all the way around (1-2-3; 1-2-3). Repeat the activity by swinging both arms backward, forward, and backward all the way around.

Part 3. Beginning with the arms hanging by the sides of the body, have the students swing the right arm diagonally up across the front of the body (1-2-3), now ask the students to swing the right arm diagonally down and out away from the right side of the body (1-2-3), now swing it down and up (in an undercurve) across the front of the body and continue swinging it up and all the way around (1-2-3; 1-2-3) in a circle (clockwise). Repeat by swinging the right arm out to the right side of the body, then swinging it across the front of the body, out to the right side again, and circle all the way around (counterclockwise). Repeat the entire pattern using the left arm.

WORD CUES the teacher can use are:

ACROSS 2 - 3, OUT 2 - 3, ACROSS 2 - 3, AROUND 2 - 3,

OUT 2 - 3, ACROSS 2 - 3, OUT 2 - 3, AROUND 2 - 3

Part 4. Beginning with the arms hanging by the sides of the body have the students swing both arms to left side (i.e. the left arm to the left side; the right arm swings across the front of the body toward the left side). Now swing both arms to the right side, and finally swing both arms to the left and all the way around (clockwise circle). Repeat the above pattern to the right side, ending with a counterclockwise circle.

Part 5. Beginning with both arms across the front of the body making the shape of an "X" with the arms, have the students swing both arms OUT, ACROSS, OUT and AROUND (arms end in an extended position parallel to the floor). Repeat by swinging the arms ACROSS, OUT, ACROSS and AROUND (arms end by making an "X" across the front of the body).

The teacher and students can create many combinations of swinging an arm or arms in a variety of directions.

ACTIVITY 2 (Swinging body parts—the legs)

Accompaniment: Music 3/4 time or counting by the teacher
Directions: (Standing in a circle with feet slightly apart and arms extended out from the sides at shoulder height and parallel to the floor)

Part 1. Instruct the students to:

Swing the right leg forward on the count of 1 - 2 - 3.
Now swing the right leg backward on the count of 1 - 2 - 3.
Now swing it forward again on the count of 1 - 2 - 3.
And step forward on the right foot on the count of 1 - 2 - 3.

Repeat this sequence using the left leg: swing forward, backward, forward, and step forward on the left foot. Repeat the sequence again with the right leg, then again with the left leg. The students will now have moved forward four steps Right, Left , Right, Left.

Part 2. Repeat the leg-swinging sequence, but begin by swinging backward, then forward, then backward, and step backward. This sequence will be performed beginning with the right leg, then the left leg, then the right leg, and finally the left leg. The students will have returned to their original starting places after the fourth backward sequence (four steps swinging forward in the pattern in Part 1 and four steps swinging backward in the pattern in Part 2).

ACTIVITY 3 (Locomotor movements—sliding)

Accompaniment: Drum
Directions: (Scattered and facing the front of the room) The following instructions can be used by the teacher:

Our locomotor warm up for today is sliding. A slide has a long and a short beat making it an uneven rhythmic pattern. (If necessary, the teacher can explain that walking is an even rhythmic pattern because every beat is the same length.) **Let us try a few sliding steps in slow motion.**

With your hands on your waist and your feet together, everyone take a step to the right side with the right foot. (This is the long or slow beat.) **Then as quickly as you can, slide your left foot over to the right foot closing your foot position and shifting the**

weight to your left foot to prepare the right foot to take the next step. (This is the short or quick beat.) (For younger students, the teacher can designate sliding toward the door or a window rather than to the right or left.)

When you step to the side, there is an open space between your feet. When you bring one foot next to the other foot, you close that space. We will use the word "step" for the leading foot which begins the slide, and "close" for the foot that immediately follows and ends the slide. One foot chases the other foot. We will take four slides, or "step-close" patterns to the right. Ready? Step (right foot) close (left foot); Step-close; Step-close; Step-close. Good everyone finished.

Another cue that the teacher can use is "step-together, step-together," instead of "step-close, step-close." Counting can also be used as a cue such as: 1 & 2 & 3 & 4 &. Count 1 is for the "step" or long beat; "&" (and) is used for the "close," "together," or the short or quick beat.

Let us use the left foot as the leader and the right foot as the follower. Get ready to step to your left with your left foot and quickly move your right foot to close the space, shifting the weight to the right foot and preparing the left foot for the next step. Ready? Step (left foot)-close (right foot); Step-close; Step-close; Step-close. (or 1 &, 2 &, 3 & 4 &, or slow-quick, slow-quick)

The teacher can repeat the sliding pattern by using the rhythmic cues of "slow-quick, slow-quick," or "long-short, long-short," as well as the Step-close cue to help the students feel the uneven rhythmic pattern of the slide.

Now that we can slide either to the right or the left sides, we will speed up the tempo. Can you slide around the room without bumping into anyone? Let us try this pattern: I will beat the drum using long-short rhythms (loud for the long beats, soft for short beats) and you will slide to the right. I may count "one-and, two-and, . . ." When the drum stops, you stop and make a shape for as long as the drum is quiet. When the drum begins you will slide to the left around the room and make another shape when the drum stops. Ready? Go.

The teacher can vary the tempo and the length of the time needed for sliding and making shapes. Depending on the time available, probably three or four repetitions will be suitable for the conclusion of the warm-ups. Following the last shape ask the students to slide to a place in the circle and sit down.

MOVEMENT EXPLORATION ACTIVITIES *(5-7 Minutes)*

ACTIVITY: "Copycat" (making your own shape; copying shapes that others make)

Accompaniment: Voice

Directions: This movement exploration activity could also be thought of as a follow-the-leader type of activity. In turn, each student creates a shape and the whole group copies the shape. From that shape, the next student creates a new shape to be copied. Copycat moves from shape to shape. The teacher should encourage the changing of levels (if everyone seems to be presenting a standing shape) by suggesting a low, medium, or high level.

(Standing in a circle) The teacher can begin Copycat by saying the following:

I am going to show you a shape and then ask you to make the same shape that I am making. Here is my shape. Everyone try this shape. Good.
(Give the student's name next to you), (Megan) **Can you change my shape to a new shape for us to copy? Good. Everyone try** (Megan's) **shape.**

Continue this activity around the circle until everyone has had a chance to make a shape and be copied. Repeat this activity around the circle at least one more time.

If a student appears to be shy or cannot seem to think of a shape, the teacher should watch carefully for the tiniest movement or shift of the body that might indicate a shape; seize that moment by copying the movement and praise the student by saying, **"Oh, that is a wonderful shape,** (student's name), **everyone try** (student's name) **shape."**

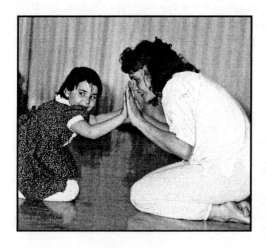

Copycat

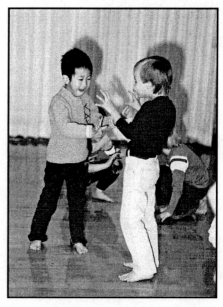

Copycat

GATHERING ACTIVITY (*10-15 Minutes*)

ACTIVITY: Build a sequence of shapes (or a shape sentence)

Accompaniment: Drum or voice; music later
Directions:

Part 1. (Standing in a circle) The teacher can use the following commentary to guide the students in this activity.

> **Everyone show me your favorite shape when I count three. Ready? One-two-three. Good. Keep that shape frozen while I have a good look at everyone's shape.**

Select four interesting, different shapes from the group. Ask each one of the four students to demonstrate his or her shape (one at a time) and have the class copy each shape. Ask the students questions about each shape such as:

What makes this shape different from another shape?
How does this shape make you feel?
Is this shape easy or difficult to make?

As a group, decide which shape will be performed first, second, third, and fourth. Repeat the shapes in the order selected to allow the students to learn and remember the shape sequence.

Part 2. (In a scattered formation) Practice the sequence of the four shapes again that were selected in Part 1. The teacher can say:

Let us see shape one. Now try shape two. What does shape three look like? Show me shape four. (Repeat the sequence one or two more times.)

Let us rest our shapes for a minute. Do you remember the swinging and sliding patterns we learned for our warm-up time? When I say go, show me one of the arm swinging patterns. (The students may present different patterns.) **Ready? Go. Good. Now, show me one of the feet sliding patterns we used. Ready? Go. Good.**

Now we are going to create a movement pattern that combines our four shapes, our arms swinging, and feet sliding.

Here is the sequence. I will give you a cue such as shape -2 - 3 - 4 , slide - 2 - 3 - 4 , or swing - 2 - 3 - 4. Each part receives four counts. Let us try the pattern.

Shape one is the beginning shape.	**Shape-2-3-4**
Slide to the right side, 4 slides.	**Slide-2-3-4**
Now make shape two.	**Shape-2-3-4**
Do the arm swings or the leg swings for 4 swings	**Swing-2-3-4**
Now make shape three.	**Shape-2-3-4**
Slide to the left side, 4 slides.	**Slide-2-3-4**
Shape four is the ending shape	**Shape-2-3-4**

Let us try this sequence together. I will tell you the movements as we go along. Show me shape one so that I will know you are ready. Good. Here we go:

Shape-2-3-4, Slide-2-3-4, Shape-2-3-4, Swing 2-3-4,
Shape-2-3-4, Slide-2-3-4, Shape-2-3-4.

Soon the teacher can stop saying the cues and allow the students to perform the sequence with some type of accompaniment. The sequence can be varied in many ways. One suggestion is to continue using 4 counts for each shape and movement but alter the sequence in the following way:

Shape #1
Slide or Swing
Shape #2
Shape #3
Swing or Slide
Shape #4

Other variations of the basic pattern can be developed by involving the students in selecting which shape to use for how many counts, what body part(s) will swing for how many counts, and which direction they will slide for how many counts.

Divide the group in half for "show and share" (performers and audience). Each performing group will show the sequence twice to its audience.

RELAXATION (5 *Minutes)*

Directions: Repeat the relaxation activities used in Lesson One, My Body Moves, or choose from the relaxation activities in Chapter 10. Younger students will enjoy the relaxation activities suggested in the story about "Kittens" in Chapter Ten (especially since this lesson focused on Copycats). Select activities that will take about 5 minutes to complete.

Time Allotment_____

Grade/Age_____

Outline of Lesson Plan Two
"Copycat"

Number of Students_____

Unit title: The Body **Lesson title:** Copycat **Date:**	**Props/Materials:** **Visual Aids:** Diagram on chalkboard Swing
Objectives 1. Explore body parts swinging 2. Explore body shapes 3. Copy shapes 4. Create a movement combination	**Equipment:** Drum, cassette/CD player **Accompaniment:** Voice, music

Activities of the Lesson	Formation	Time
WARM UPS 1. arm swings 2. leg swings 3. slides - right + left	Standing Scattered	5 min.
MOVEMENT EXPLORATION ACTIVITIES Follow-the-leader – copy shapes Explore levels + shapes Repeat activity	Circle: Standing	5-7 min.
GATHERING ACTIVITY 1. Show favorite shape - select shapes from 4 students, try each shape - class decides order of 4 shapes = 1-2-3-4 and perform pattern 2. Pattern combination: Shape 1 + slide right Shape 2 + swing Shape 3 + slide left 3. Show + Share Shape 4 = ending	Circle: Standing Scattered	10-15 min.
RELAXATION Repeat activities from Lesson one "My Body Moves" Chapter 10 "Kittens"	Circle: Sitting lying on back	5 min
Evaluation of the lesson: 1. What went well? 2. What can be improved?		

QUESTIONS TEACHERS CAN ASK STUDENTS ABOUT THE BODY

These sample questions are designed to assist the teacher in guiding the students in exploring body movement. Teachers will soon develop a long list of questions that will challenge students and provide enjoyable and successful experiences for everyone.

1. How may different ways can you move your _____? (name a body part: head, toes, arms, legs . . .)
2. Can you move two body parts in the same direction?
3. Can you move two body parts in different directions?
4. How many different shapes can you make with your arm(s), leg(s), shoulders, (or other body parts)?
5. How many different shapes can you make with your whole body?
6. Can you make a shape at a high, medium, or low level?
7. Can you make a shape and move it to another part of the room?
8. What kind of shapes can you make with a partner?

The following phrases stimulate students to action without being told the exact movement to make. These phrases will work with any lessons in this book, or any lessons that teachers develop as a result of methods and techniques used in this book. The phrases solicit the best performance a student can offer at the moment.

1. How many different ways . . .?
2. Can you . . .?
3. Show me . . .
4. Show me a new way to . . .
5. What kind of action or shape can you . . .?
6. Try . . .(the teacher suggests a movement task such as a shape with an elbow and a knee touching)

As the teacher becomes more skilled in posing these types of challenges, new combinations of questions will develop.

BODY WORDS FOR MOVEMENT EXPLORATION

Often a word or a phrase can provide ideas for creative movement activities. This section is intended to assist the teacher with words and exercises related to developing lessons concerning the body. The following words relate to body parts, shapes, positions, combinations, and actions.

1. **Whole Body**

2. **Body Parts**

head	spine	wrists	feet
neck	hips	fingers	heels
shoulders	arms	thumbs	ankles
chest	lower arms	legs	toes
waist	upper arms	thighs	stomach
elbows	shins	knees	back
hands			

3. **Combinations of Body Parts**

elbows/knees	shoulders/hips
arms/legs	hands/feet
hands /knees	trunk/head

4. **Body Shapes**

curved	angular	straight
twisted	narrow	wide

5. **Geometric Shapes to Make with the Body or Body Parts**

round	triangle
triangle	rectangle

6. **Body Surfaces**

front	back	side

7. **Body Positions**

   lying (front, back, side)

sitting	kneeling	standing

8. **Body Movement**

   a. **Nonlocomotor** (performed on a stationary base—in place)

bend	dodge	push
twist	strike	pull
stretch	fall	rock
sway	rise	lift
swing	turn	shake

   (continued)

b. Locomotor (performed on a moving base—traveling)

<u>Even rhythm</u>	<u>Uneven rhythm</u>
walk	skip
run	slide
hop	gallop
leap	
jump	

c. Combinations of Nonlocomotor Actions

alone-together	stretching-bending
swinging-swaying	twisting-turning
rocking-rolling	shaking-freezing
tensing-collapsing	rising-falling
pushing-pulling	alternating

A MOVEMENT EXPLORATION ACTIVITY
FOR THE BODY

Teachers can read the following activity to the students, (adapting the phrasing as necessary) and have them explore "Body Wheels." Pictures of machinery using wheels (or actual machinery) can serve as a visual aid for introducing this activity. A scattered formation is suggested for beginning the activity individually, followed by the students selecting partners, and finally the whole class will move together. Teachers can adapt this activity to their students and use any one or all of these suggested groupings.

As soon as the students have explored "Body Wheels," they may be able to think of ways to extend this activity by adding props such as elastic bands, cardboard tubes, or machinery parts that could be incorporated into the movement sequence. The students may also create another movement activity based on their experiences of exploring "Body Wheels."

Body Wheels by *Jean Warren* (1984)

How many ways can your children make wheels with their bodies? Can they make their heads turn like wheels? Their arms, hands, fingers, hips, legs, feet? Can they make more than one body wheel move at a time? In different directions?

Have the children pair up and coordinate their bodies in some way to make a machine that runs on wheels—as many wheels as possible.

(continued)

As a grand finale, have all the children come together and create one giant machine made up of many wheels and moving parts. All the wheels can work together simultaneously, or one wheel can begin turning, activate the next wheel, and so on until all the wheels are turning. As the last wheel turns, the machine can "Bong!" and wind down by having the wheels slow down and stop in reverse order (p. 79).

CHANTS FOR BODY PARTS

The following chants were used by permission from the author, Ann Zirulnik (1979). She stated that "chants are fun, easy to remember, and reinforce vocabulary." She suggested choosing "one of the chants for the day [and] for the next lesson, you might repeat today's chant and add a new one." Chants can be used for warm ups, movement exploration activities, or the gathering activity. Quiet, slow chants can be created for relaxation activities to end a lesson. Some of Zurulnik's (1979) chants are:

Shake your hand and hop around (Keep the action going and add on)
Shake your head and hop around
Shake your leg and hop around
Jump - Jump - Jump
[other locomotor movements and body parts can be substituted for the ones in the chant such as: shake your arm and skip around.]

Put your hands in the air
Put your hands in your hair (Keep hands here)
Move your body everywhere.

(Sitting down, legs out in front)
Touch your fingers to your toes
Touch your fingers to your nose
Touch your fingers to your knees
Twirl around, if you please. [*spin around on the seat or feet*]

Walk in a circle
Walk in a line
Walk in a zig zag
Stop on a dime.

(*continued*)

> I'm jumping in place
> And make a funny face
> I'm sitting on the ground
> And turning all around.
>
> Clap your hands
> Stomp your feet
> Wiggle your back and
> Show your teeth.
>
> Now I'm high and
> Now I'm low
> Now I'm fast and
> Now I'm slow (p.6)

Vary these chants by performing them at different speeds. You can ask the students to do the chant in their own tempo and to make changes based upon their experimention. Students can also make up their own chants such as:

> I have two hands and I have two feet
> I have one face that is very sweet.

They can then share their chants with the class, make up movements to go with the chant, and have the class perform them.

SUMMARY

This chapter presented two lessons concerning the element of the body. **Lesson One, My Body Moves,** explored movement of different body parts. A shape-movement-shape sequence was developed as a gathering activity. **Lesson Two, Copycat,** emphasized making shapes with the body and copying the shapes that others created. The gathering activity suggested that the teacher select four shapes created by four students and build a pattern for class participation using a beginning, a middle, and an ending which included these shapes along with the sliding and swinging activities.

Body words for movement exploration, a movement exploration activity, "Body Wheels," and chants for body parts were included at the end of the chapter as resources for the teacher. These activities can be used to enhance the sample lessons as well as create new lessons based on the element of the body. The chapter ended with The Idea Page which provides a place for teachers to write ideas for future lessons, or ideas for activities that can be used within lessons they plan to create.

THE IDEA PAGE

Chapter 5

TIME

INTRODUCTION

This chapter focuses on the element of **time**. The components of time related to movement consist of:

Tempo	—	the speed of the music or movement (slow to fast)
Beat	—	a measurement of time regardless of the tempo (underlying beat like a heart beat)
Accent	—	movement more forceful than the movement preceding or following it; (as in music where the additional emphasis may be placed on a certain pulse or beat in a series)
Duration	—	the length of each beat or movement (short or long)
Rhythmic Pattern	—	a succession of movements or sounds of varying duration (also includes tempo, beat and accent)

Within this chapter, two lessons will be presented which focus on the concepts of time, yet build upon the body concepts addressed in Chapter 4. The teacher may use these lessons as beginning points, but should move toward modifying them and creating new lessons which are directly related to his or her own students and classes.

OBJECTIVES

1. To move body parts fast and slow
2. To move in space fast and slow
3. To create a fast and slow movement pattern
4. To create a pattern

WARM-UPS (5 Minutes)

ACTIVITY 1

Accompaniment: Voices of teacher and students

Directions: (Sitting in a circle with legs stretched forward) Use Warm-Up Activity 1 "Head and shoulders, knees and toes" in Lesson One, Chapter 4. Either chant or sing the words using the tune of "London Bridge is Falling Down." To explore a slow and fast tempo, the following sequence is suggested:

1. Perform the entire chant (both parts) very slowly as a review and also to provide a contrast for a coming change in tempo.
2. Perform the entire chant as fast as possible without mixing up the words or omitting body parts.
3. Perform the first part of the chant (head, shoulders, knees, toes) very fast and the second part (eyes, ears, nose, chin) very slowly.
4. Allow the students to perform the chant at their own tempo.

ACTIVITY 2

Accompaniment: Drum

Directions: (Standing in a scattered formation) Have the students walk around the room taking one step with each drum beat and speed up or slow down with the drum. Remind the students that they are to avoid bumping into anyone and that when the drum stops they are to stop. The following sequence can be used or varied:

1. Begin slowly and increase the tempo until the students are walking quickly. Stop the drum beat. The students stop.
2. Begin with a fast tempo and slow down to a very slow beat until the drum stops and the students stop.
3. The tempo of the walk (or another locomotor movement) can be varied along with the direction in which the students travel.

Beat a fast tempo for a short duration and stop; beat a slow tempo for a long duration and stop; or choose another combination to challenge the students as they warm-up.

MOVEMENT EXPLORATION ACTIVITIES (5-7 *Minutes*)

The following activities are suggested for adding the element of *time* to the teaching of creative movement. As the following activities are explored, make sure that the students are given enough time to experiment with the suggested movements. Teachers should feel free to change the sample to suit their classroom structures and styles of teaching.

Part 1. (Sitting in a circle) The teacher can say:

Everyone shake your right hand as fast as you can, freeze, and relax that hand. Now move your right hand just as slowly as you can. Good. Try shaking your left hand as fast as you can. Ready? Go. Freeze, relax, and now move your left hand as slowly as possible. What other body part can you move fast? Ready? Go. Show me another body part and how slowly it can move. Good.

Part 2. (Standing in a circle) The teacher may say:

Everyone stand up and show me a body part that can move fast while you are standing still. Good. Try moving a body part very slowly while you are standing on one leg. Very good balancing. Can you move one body part fast while you are moving another body part slowly? Try it now. Can you make a quick, sudden movement with your whole body when I beat the drum? Ready? (Beat the drum, or clap once. Repeat the sudden-movement activity several times encouraging the students to use different body parts, shapes, and levels.)

When I beat the gong (or make a vocal sound of "shhhhhh" that gradually decreases in volume) **show me a slow movement that goes on until you cannot hear the sound any more. Ready?** (Beat the gong or use your voice.) **Try this slow motion movement with another body part** (gong or voice accompanies); **the whole body** (gong or voice); **and one more body part** (gong or voice). **Good.**

This time show me a shape that changes slowly from a high to a low level when you hear the gong (or voice). Good for you. When you hear a drum beat only *once,* change from the low level where you are now to a high level as fast as you can. Ready? (Beat the drum once or clap once.) (Repeat this activity moving quickly or slowly to various levels. Allow the students to select their own levels and tempo a few times).

How many of you think you can walk slowly around the room without bumping into anyone? Good, let us try. When the drum (or clapping) begins, start walking forward around the room. (The teacher can select a clockwise or counterclockwise direction, or allow the students to choose.) When the drum stops, what do you do? (Wait for an answer.) Freeze, that is right. Ready? Begin. (Allow the students to walk slowly throughout the room.) Freeze. Can you walk very fast around the room without bumping into anyone? Ready? Go. Freeze. Do you think you can run without bumping into anyone? Remember to stop when the drum stops. Ready? Go. (Allow the students to run throughout the room as long as they are moving safely among each other.) Freeze and sit down right where you are.

GATHERING ACTIVITY *(10-15 Minutes)*

Part 1. After the students have experimented with the various exploration activities, begin to assemble the activities into patterns as follows:

We are going to combine moving your body through space, stopping, and making a shape." (Each pattern contains a locomotor movement, a stop, and making a shape in place.) Let me see if you can walk, stop, and make a shape. Be careful not to bump into anyone. Ready? Go. Walk (beat the drum or clap for a walking pattern), stop, shape. Good (if the students managed to move without bumping into anyone). Try that combination again. Ready? Go. Good. This time try walking slowly, stopping, making a shape and slowly changing that shape while staying in one place. Ready? Go. Walk, stop, shape, and now change the shape slowly in place. (Repeat this sequence a few times.)

Now we are changing the pattern so that you will walk very quickly and make a shape and quickly change that shape to another shape while staying in one place . Ready? Go. Good. (Repeat this pattern again.)

For the gathering activity the teacher and students can make many combinations of locomotor movements (fast or slow) and shapes (fast or slow). For example: run, stop, and make a shape slowly , or run, stop, and make a shape as fast as possible. Repeat the pattern and make a shape in place that has a slow or fast moving body part.

Part 2. Explore combinations of the fast and slow sequences. The *fast* pattern is *run,* stop, make a fast moving shape in place. The *slow* pattern is *walking slowly,* stop, make a slowly moving shape in place. Alternate the movement patterns so that each group will perform four patterns. Begin with a fast, slow, fast, slow combination. Other combinations of the fast, slow patterns can be varied in the following ways: fast, fast, slow, slow; slow, fast, fast, slow; or other combinations can be suggested by the students. Incorporate making a shape quickly or slowly that freezes; then a shape that stays in place but has a fast or slow moving part.

Divide the class into two groups—performers and audience—and have each group perform for the other.

RELAXATION *(5 Minutes)*

(Standing in a circle) Have the students reach their arms toward the ceiling. The teacher can give the following instructions:

See if you can stretch so high that you almost touch the ceiling. Gently keep stretching one arm up and then the other arm reaching as high as you can. Now bring your arms down slowly to your shoulders, to your waist, to your knees, and touch the floor. Stay bending over for a moment and let your arms hang long and feel heavy. Now slowly begin to straighten up and reach for the ceiling once more—stretching, reaching with each arm. Slowly bend over and touch the floor with your fingers and gradually straighten up and reach to the ceiling.

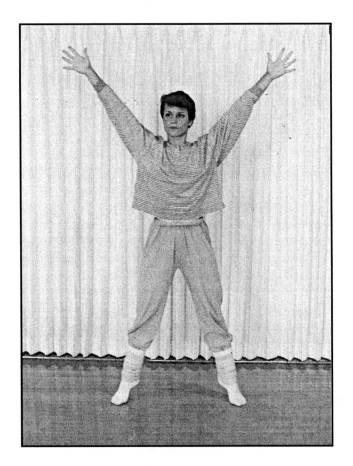

Reaching

From the reaching-to-the-ceiling position have the students slowly "melt" to the floor like ice cream in the hot sun. Have the students stretch out on the floor on their backs with their arms next to their sides, legs together and straight on the floor, and eyes closed. Play slow, quiet music for about one minute (or longer if time permits). When the music stops have the students stretch their arms and legs while they are still lying on the floor. Then have the students slowly sit up and rise to a standing position. Use movement tasks to take the students to their socks and shoes.

Outline of Lesson Plan One
"How Do I Move"

	Props/Materials:
Unit title: *Time* Lesson title: *How Do I Move?* Date:	**Visual Aids:**
Objectives 1. move body parts fast + slow 2. move through space fast + slow 3. create a movement pattern	Equipment: *Drum, Gong cassette/CD player* **Accompaniment:** *Voice percussion, music*

Activities of the Lesson	Formation	Time
WARM UPS 1. Chant: head, shoulders, knees + toes - use different tempos 2. Walking: slow to fast, fast to slow	Circle: Sitting Standing Scattered	5 min.
MOVEMENT EXPLORATION ACTIVITIES 1. Shake + freeze body parts 2. In place - move body parts fast + slow 3. Combine fast + slow movements with levels 4. Walk, run at different tempos	Circle: Standing Scattered	5-7 min
GATHERING ACTIVITY COMBINATIONS: (move, stop, shape) 1. Walk, stop, shape (regular tempo) 2. Walk, stop, shape (slow/fast tempos) 3. Run, stop, make shape slowly - repeat 4. Run stop, make shape fast - repeat F = Fast: run, stop - FAST moving shape S: Slow: walk, stop - SLOW moving shape Explore: FSFS - FFSS - SFFS. Show + Share	Standing Scattered	10-15min
RELAXATION 1. Stretch to ceiling, bend - touch toes 2. "melt" 3. Lie quietly, stretch + relax 4. Listen to music, eyes closed, relaxed body	Standing Collapse Lying on back	5 min.
Evaluation of the lesson: 1. What went well? 2. What can be improved?		

OBJECTIVES

1. To explore body movements in relationship to musical note values (whole, half, quarter, eighth notes)
2. To explore body shapes in relationship to musical note values
3. To create a locomotor pattern based on the musical note values in 4/4 time (whole, half, quarter, eighth notes)
4. To incorporate visual aids with the movement activity

WARM-UPS *(5 Minutes)*

ACTIVITY 1

Accompaniment: Music with a steady beat of 4 or 8 counts
Directions: (Standing in circle) Use the sequence in Warm-Up Activity 1, Part 2 in Lesson One of Chapter 4. The cues the teacher can use for this warm-up are:

Stretch 2 - 3 - 4 - 5 - 6 - 7 - 8
Bend elbows and knees 2 - 3 - 4
Hang and shake 2 - 3 - 4
Uncurl slowly (straighten knees) 2 - 3 - 4, (back) 5 - 6, (neck) 7, (head) 8.

Repeat the sequence using a fast tempo for the arm stretches and a slow tempo for the remainder of the sequence. Experiment with varying the tempo.

ACTIVITY 2

Accompaniment: Music with a steady beat of 4 or 8 counts
Directions:

Part 1. (Sitting in circle, arms and legs crossed) Have the students twist as far as they can around to the right side using 4 counts and twist to the left side using 4 counts.
Repeat this sequence slowly two more times.

Part 2. (In a squatting or sitting position facing the center of the circle) Have the students twist upwards to the right, and continue turning and rising until they are standing, facing the center of the circle. Use 8 counts for this part of the sequence. Next, have the students twist to the left and continue turning and lowering themselves until they have reached the squatting or sitting position from which they began. Use 8 counts for this part of the pattern. This movement could be thought of (or visualized) as a spiral upward and downward. This activity is challenging to students to test their skills in rising and sitting without using their hands.

ACTIVITY 3

Accompaniment: March music with a steady beat
Directions: (Scattered formation, standing) Have the students march around the room (either clockwise or counterclockwise). When the music stops, the students will stop. The following sequence is suggested for the teacher to use. Have the students:

> March forward around the room, stop when the music stops, and make a shape.
> March backward around the room, stop when the music stops, and make a shape.
> March forward and clap hands with each step, stop in place when the music stops.
> March backward and clap hands with each step, stop in place when the music stops.

MOVEMENT EXPLORATION ACTIVITIES *(5-7 Minutes)*

(Sitting in a group facing the teacher) Show the students a picture of a whole note, a half note, a quarter note, and an eighth note (based on information in Figure 2). Explain how many counts each note receives for a 4/4 time signature. Explain the *sound* that each note makes.

The teacher may introduce this lesson to the students by using the following words:

I will show you a picture of the musical notes that we are going to learn. Each note has a certain number of counts and lasts a certain length of time. Look at the poster with the notes and the counts. (Show a poster or create an overhead transparency based on Figure 3.)

The star indicates that a sound should be made and followed by the number of beats indicated. In the case of a whole note, a sound would be made on the first beat and held for three additional beats. The half notes in the figure indicate that for two

half notes a sound is made on the first beat and held for the second beat of that note. And for the second half note of the measure (as indicated in Figure 3) a sound would be made on the third beat and held on the fourth beat.

Let us clap the sound we should hear for each note. For notes that have more than one count, keep your hands together and move your hands slightly downward in a pulse for each count—only our voices will be heard saying the number. Let us try our clapping and counting as we identify the various notes.

Musical Note Values

		Number of Notes to make 4 counts	Counts per note	Sounds per measure
Whole note	o	1	4	1
Half note	♩	2	2	2
Quarter note	♩	4	1	4
Eighth note	♪	8	1/2	8

Whole = one note; 4 counts per note   o

Half = two notes; 2 counts per note   ♩   ♩

Quarter = four notes; 1 count per note   ♩ ♩ ♩ ♩

Eighth = eight notes; 1/2 count per note   ♪ ♪ ♪ ♪ ♪ ♪ ♪ ♪

Figure 2

Basic Rhythmic Pattern of 4/4 Time

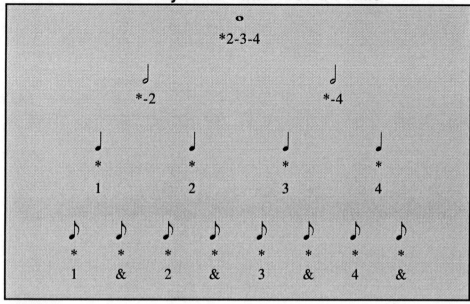

Figure 3

Foot Pattern for Basic Rhythmic Pattern in 4/4 Time

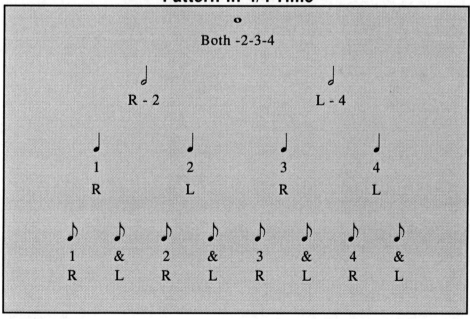

Figure 4

The teacher and students should count out loud 4 counts for each measure, and clap or tap their feet for the sound each note receives. As the sound pattern is learned ask the students to stop counting out loud and just let their clapping and pulsing movements keep the rhythm.

For a further challenge of this rhythmic activity, the teacher may want to try combining the pattern with clapping hands and tapping feet, first in a sitting position, then standing in place, and finally moving around the room. The students can test their balance and coordination with this activity.

One idea is to create a series of four-count measures. The first measure could be a whole note with one movement held for 4 counts. The second measure could be two half notes with one movement for each note; each movement held for 2 counts. The third measure could be made of four quarter notes with one movement for each note; each movement held for 1 count.

GATHERING ACTIVITY *(10-15 Minutes)*

Present the following pattern to the students by using a poster or overhead transparency of the notes and rhythmic patterns so that they can learn to recognize the different kinds of notes and also see a relationship between the note values and the movement selected. One idea is to create a series of four-count measures. The first measure could be a whole note with one movement held for 4 counts. The second measure could be two half notes with one movement for each note; each movement held for 2 counts. The third measure could be made of four quarter notes with one movement for each note; each movement held for 1 count. This idea could be extended to creating 8 movements (which would need to be small and quick) for an eighth note. (Make the poster based on the rhythmic pattern in Figure 5 and use Figure 6 for a variation of the rhythmic pattern.) Remember the concept that a slow tempo allows more time to move and larger movements can be performed, while a fast tempo reduces the time to move and smaller movements are required.

A Rhythmic Movement Pattern

	walk	walk	run a lit- tle		slow	down	stop	
4/4	♩	♩	♪ ♪ ♪ ♪		♩	♩	o	
	1	2	3 & 4 &		1-2	3-4	1-2-3-4	
	R	L	R L R L		R	L	R	

Figure 5

A Variation of a Rhythmic Movement Pattern

	slow	down	walk	walk	run	a	lit-	tle	stop
4/4	♩	♩	♩	♩	♪	♪	♪	♪	o
	1-2	3-4	1	2	3	&	4	&	1-2-3-4
	R	L	R	L	R	L	R	L	R

Figure 6

The musical and movement pattern in Figures 5 and 6 consists of three measures of 4 beats each. The time signatures in Figures 5 and 6 are 4/4. The first number (which also appears in some music as the top number) indicates the number of beats per measure—in this case, 4 beats per measure. The second number after the stroke line (or the bottom number in musical notation) indicates the type of note that receives 1 beat or count—in this case, the quarter note receives 1 count.

Show the students the poster of the pattern that includes the notes, counts, and locomotor movements. Have the students clap the rhythm of the pattern and try the steps while sitting. Then ask the students to stand and find their own places in the room. The teacher may explain the pattern in the following way:

> **Our pattern will be two walks. Each walk will receive 1 count. Next we have four little runs. Each step of the run will receive 1/2 count each. The word "slow" gets 2 counts and the word "Down" gets 2 counts. "Stop" is a whole note and receives 4 counts. Let us try this pattern. I will clap and tell you the movements as you go through the pattern. Here we go.**

Walk	Walk	run	a	lit - tle	
1	2	3	&	4	&

Slow		Down		
1	2	3		4

Stop				
1	2	3		4

The following sequence could be used to develop the gathering activity:

1. Repeat the pattern a few times in a forward direction and increase the tempo with each repetition to locate the proper speed for the skill of the students.
2. Try the pattern with the students walking backwards making sure no one bumps into anyone.
3. Next have the students try one pattern walking forward and then one pattern walking backward.
4. Now, add three shape patterns with 4 counts for each shape pattern (standing in place) between the forward and backward pattern. Each shape pattern could be treated as a whole note—on the count of "one" the students make a shape and hold that shape for counts "2-3-4."
5. (For a further challenge, Shape Pattern 1 could be treated as quarter notes with one movement in place for each count, Shape Pattern 2 could be two half notes that require two movements (one movement each on counts "1"and "3"), and Shape Pattern 3 could be treated as a whole note with one movement. Many combinations could be developed. The whole pattern would then be:

Forward (one complete pattern of walk, walk, run a little, slow down, stop)

Shape Pattern 1 (4 counts)	one shape on count 1 and hold for 3 counts (total 1 shape)
Shape Pattern 2 (4 counts)	one shape on count 1 and hold for 1 count, one shape on count 3 and hold for 1 count (total 2 shapes)
Shape Pattern 3 (4 counts)	one shape for each count (total of 4 shapes)

Backward (one complete pattern of walk, walk, run a little, slow down, stop).

Shape Pattern 3 (4 counts) = 4 shapes
Shape Pattern 2 (4 counts) = 2 shapes (on counts 1 & 3)
Shape Pattern 1 (4 counts) = 1 shape

If the shapes in the above lesson are varied according to the note values, students can make their own choices about which shape will equal a certain note value. The accompanying or underlying beat would continue to be the basic 4-count measure. The movements of the students, however, will add variety and interest because some students will choose a whole-note shape and make one movement for Shape Pattern 1, while other students may choose a quarter-note shape and make four movements during that same Shape Pattern 1.

As a closing to the gathering activity, divide the class into the accompanists and the performers. The performers will present the pattern that was created in step 4 (above) using each shape as a whole note with just one movement per shape, while the accompanists clap a total of six measures of 4 beats each. Have the students perform the pattern twice and then trade groups. To keep track of the measures as they are counted and performed, the counting can be: 1-2-3-4; (measure two) 2-2-3-4; (measure three) 3-2-3-4; (measure four) 4-2-3-4; (measure five) 5-2-3-4; and (measure six) 6-2-3-4.

This lesson *particularly* provides opportunities to incorporate mathematics into the creative movement activity. Students can be asked how many measures there are in the basic pattern? How many total counts are in a basic pattern? Other mathematical questions will be formulated as the teacher develops further lessons.

RELAXATION (5 *Minutes*)

Have the students lie down on their backs with their legs together, stretched long and their arms resting on the floor extended above their heads. Use slow music, and while the music is playing ask the students to:

Stretch your RIGHT arm and your RIGHT leg in opposite directions as far as you can, then relax.
Repeat this action with your LEFT arm and LEFT leg and relax.

Now try stretching your RIGHT arm and your LEFT leg as far as you can, then relax.
Finally, try stretching your LEFT arm and your RIGHT leg in opposite directions, and relax.

Stretch BOTH arms and BOTH legs as far as you can in the opposite directions, reach, reach, and relax.

With all body parts relaxed, close your eyes and breathe slowly in through the nose (inhale) and then out through the mouth (exhale) as the music plays.

Allow the students to rest in this position and gradually lower the volume of the music until it is no longer heard. Then instruct the students to sit up slowly, stretch, and stand up. Use movement tasks to have the students put on their socks and shoes.

Outline of Lesson Plan Two
"The Beat Goes On"

Unit title: *Time* **Lesson title:** *The Beat Goes On* **Date:**	**Props/Materials:** **Visual Aids:** *Charts*	
Objectives 1. *relate body movements + musical note values* 2. " " *shapes* " " " " 3. *create a pattern*	**Equipment:** *Drum,* *cassette / CD player* **Accompaniment:** *Voice,* *percussion, music*	

Activities of the Lesson	Formation	Time
WARM UPS 1. *Stretch, bend, "hangover," curl up* 2. *Slow twists side-to-side, rise up + lower down* 3. *Marching - forward, backward* *add - hand clap with march step*	*Circle:* *Sitting* *Standing* *Scattered*	*5 min.*

MOVEMENT EXPLORATION ACTIVITIES
 Use Charts
    Sounds - Counting, moving, freezing
    Chart 1 - Hand Clap
    Chart 2 - Feet tap
	Sitting
	 group facing
	 teacher
		5-7 min.

GATHERING ACTIVITY
 Explore rhythmic pattern with words
    at levels of (1) sitting, (2) standing, (3) moving
 Explore Variation
 Combine pattern with variation (use different
    directions - forward, backward, etc.)
 Show + Share
	Sit
	 Stand
	
	 Scattered
		10-15 min

RELAXATION *Stretch arms, legs, alternate R + L* *Breathing ; Close eyes + relax all over* *Slow music - find quiet inner self*	*Lying on back*	*5 min*
Evaluation of the lesson: 1. What went well? 2. What can be improved?		

QUESTIONS TEACHERS CAN ASK STUDENTS ABOUT TIME

Riggs (1980) suggested the following questions that can assist the teacher in guiding students through creative movement experiences.

> How do I move? [in relationship to time]?
> How fast or slowly can I move?
> Can I move as though I am in slow motion?
> Can I make a movement go on and on slowly for a long time?
> What is the most sudden movement I can make with my whole body?
> Or with one arm? Or with my feet?
> Can I change from doing quick, sudden movements to slow ones?
> (p. 10)

TIME WORDS FOR MOVEMENT EXPLORATION

This section is intended to assist the teacher with "time" materials related to developing lessons concerning the exploration of this element. The following words may provide ideas for creative movement activities. The teacher and students will be able to add to this list.

fast	medium	sudden
regular	irregular	slow
even	uneven	quick
long	short	

The following poem also combines the elements of time and space providing many movement words and ideas that can be used as a part of a lesson in the warm ups, movement exploration activities, or the gathering activities.

While the students sit in a circle, the teacher asks them to **listen** for movement words, and to **think** about ways they might move as the poem is read for the first time. Then have the students move into a scattered formation and the teacher will read the poem the second time giving the students time to create shapes and movements as they hear the "movement words."

Contrasts In Time and Space (Elf to Giant)

Slowly grow up toward the sky
As thin and straight as you are high
Slowly curl and twist yourself
Going downwards like an elf ....
You're two inches tall!

Quickly, shoot up tall and thin,
Slowly down to [the] floor again ....

Slowly toward the ceiling go,
Now quickly twisting, down you go!

Stretch arms and body outward, narrow.
Until you look quite like an arrow
Bring yourself back straight again
Stand quite slender, like a pen.
Crumple down, into a ball—
You hardly need a space at all!

Up! Now, like a giant tall
Looking out on rooftops all
One hand sweeps the tops of trees
While the other skims the breeze.

Sweep, and skim, and take big strides
(But no one with a giant collides!)
For if two giants touch at all
It breaks the spell - and that is ALL!. . . . (Gong) (p. 31)

by special permission of Grace C. Nash, author. From
Verses and Movement, Grace Nash Publications,
Scottsdale, Arizona 85252, U.S.A.

SUMMARY

The concept of time and its relationship to movement was explored in the two sample lessons presented in this chapter. Some of the terms used were: tempo, beat, accent, duration, and rhythmic patterns.

Lesson One, How Do I Move?, explored fast and slow tempos of movement with body parts and moving the body through space. The lesson culminated in movement patterns of a fast locomotor movement plus making a shape as quickly as possible, and then making a shape in place with a body part that moves fast. A contrasting sequence using slow movements was created.

Lesson Two, The Beat Goes On, explored ways in which movement and musical note values relate. A rhythmic movement pattern was developed that used whole, half, quarter, and eighth notes with walking, running, slowing down, and stopping.

Additional resource materials from which the teacher can develop further lessons included questions teachers can ask students about time and time words (including poetry) for movement exploration. The Idea Page ends this chapter to allow space for the ideas the teacher has discovered for future lessons.

ADVENTURES IN CREATIVE MOVEMENT ACTIVITIES

THE IDEA PAGE

Chapter 6

SPACE

INTRODUCTION

Space is an important element of movement and contains several parts which are used in creative movement activities. Space is concerned with the following aspects:

Personal Space — the space that immediately surrounds an individual. It extends as far as one can reach in any direction from a stationary position. Personal space accompanies the individual everywhere. It is sometimes referred to as self space.

General Space — the space in which movement takes place — a classroom, multi-purpose room, or gymnasium. A mover travels from one place to another in general space. It is sometimes referred to as environmental space.

Direction — forward, backward, sideward, diagonal, up, down

Level — high, medium, low

(continued)

Range (size)	— near to, far from (big, little)
Pathways	— curved, straight, angular (patterns on the floor or in the air)
Shape	— angular, circular, straight
Focus	— direction in which the eyes are looking

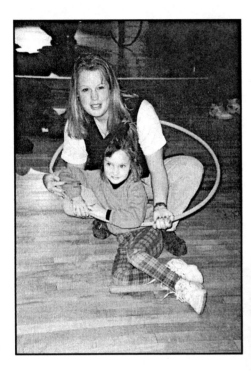

**Curved Shapes
at a Low Level**

Combination: Straight, Angular and Curved Shape at a Middle Level

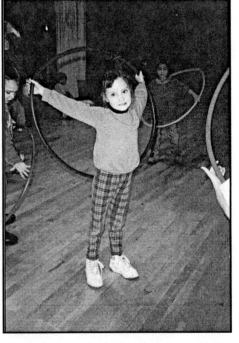

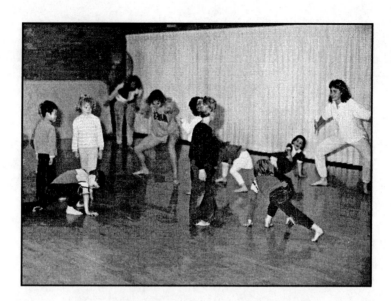

Angular Shapes at Different Levels

This chapter focuses on the element of space and its relationship to movement. Two sample lessons are described that explore moving in personal space and moving through general space. While space is the main element explored in these two lessons, the body is the instrument using time and force to explore the spatial aspects of movement. Resource information at the end of the chapter provides questions for the teacher to ask students about space, and "space words" for movement exploration. A poem, "Walking in Space," offers ideas for developing new creative movement lessons.

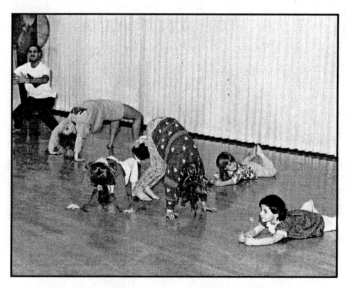

Circular Shape at Different Levels

LESSON ONE—MY PLACE IN SPACE

OBJECTIVES

1. To explore personal space
2. To explore general space
3. To explore direction and levels
4. To create a pattern combining all parts of the lesson

WARM-UPS *(5 Minutes)*

ACTIVITY 1

Accompaniment: Poem "Contrasts in Space"
Directions: (Students sitting in a circle with legs crossed and hands in laps.) Have the students explore their personal space by reaching their arms forward, backward, upward, downward, and to the sides (right arm to right side; left arm to left side) reaching as far as their arms can extend.

(Students standing) Repeat this exercise and challenge students to see if they can reach further than when they were sitting. The students may discover that they can reach a little further by bending the body forward, backward, or to the side, or by stepping one foot out in any direction. Have the students find their own places in the room and sit down. Make sure that they are not touching anyone and that they have plenty of space around them.

Read the following poem while the students listen. Then, read the poem again and have students interpret it through movement.

Suggestions for movement are in parentheses prior to each line of the poem, in case some students need assistance. Other students will think of different acceptable ways to move to this poetry.

Contrasts In Space

(reach up)
How high is the <u>ceiling</u>?- - -up, up, up (reach on tiptoes)

(reach down)
How low is the <u>floor</u>? - - - -reach, down, down

(stretch out)
How far goes the ocean?- - -arms out

(pull in)
How in is a <u>pin</u>? - - - -body in, in, in
ceiling....floor....ocean....pin. (p. 10)

by special permission of Grace C. Nash, author. From
Verses and Movement, Grace C. Nash Publications,
Scottsdale, Arizona 85252, U.S.A.

ACTIVITY 2

Accompaniment: Drum
Directions: (Standing in a scattered formation) Locomotor movements
require space. This activity uses the movements of leaping to move through
horizontal space and jumping to move in vertical space. Draw a circle on
the board with a horizontal line through the middle. The top half of the
circle is the path of a leap.

Part 1. Begin by having the students walk around the room, then ask them
to take longer steps until those steps become leaps. Suggest that they leap
over imaginary obstacles, such as a ditch or a log, alternating feet as they
leap covering the widest distance possible. Use a drum to accompany a
leap pattern of eight leaps with students alternating feet. Stop and rest.
Challenge the students to leap as far as they can without bumping into
anyone. Repeat eight leaps, stop, and rest.

Part 2. Next have the students **practice** jumping. There are three parts to
a jump: (a) the preparation, (b) the jump, and (c) the return or recovery
from the jump. Have the students begin by bending their knees (in ballet
this movement is called a plie [plee-ay]) in preparation for the jump,
straighten the knees pretending to take off in the air, and then bend the
knees (plie) again on the return from "outer space." Students should be
taking off with two feet and landing with two feet.

Part 3. As soon as the technique of careful, safe jumping is completed,
have the students cover vertical space by jumping as high as they can once,
then twice, and three times, stop, and rest. When you beat the drum they
will jump on each beat. Finally, have the students jump five times
consecutively (beat the drum to accompany them), stop, and rest. Make
sure that the students bend their knees to cushion the landing following
each jump.

Part 4. Combine walking, leaping, and jumping into a short movement pattern. A suggested pattern is 8 walking steps in a small circle, 8 leaps forward, 4 jumps in place, and 4 counts to rest. Then repeat the pattern one more time to complete the warm-up activities.

MOVEMENT EXPLORATION ACTIVITIES *(5-7 Minutes)*

(Standing in a circle with each student an arm's distance apart. Students face the center of the circle and extend their arms straight out from their shoulders to each side and touch only the fingertips of the students on each side.)

Part 1. The teacher can give the following directions:

In the space where you are standing, show me how many different directions your body parts can stretch. We will begin with the head first. Now the shoulders, arms, elbows, hands and fingers, chest, stomach, hips, legs, knees, feet, and toes.

Name each body part separately and have the students explore the different directions in which each body part can stretch or reach before going on to the next body part.

Part 2. Continue the lesson by giving the following instructions:

Let us try a shape that uses *one* body part stretching out in *one* direction. Try stretching *two* body parts in the *same* direction. Can you stretch *two* body parts in *different* directions?

Now try stretching *two* body parts in the *same* direction and *one* body part in a *different* direction.
Think about tree branches and all of the different directions the branches stretch out. Can you branch out in many directions with many body parts?

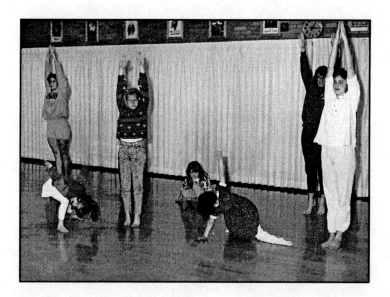

Stretching Two Body Parts in Different Directions

Part 3. Adding a change of level to the "branching" activity can challenge the skills and imagination of the students. The teacher can continue the exploration activity with these directions:

> **During the warm ups you jumped and leaped and those movements changed your level in space. Let us see if you can change levels with your whole body. Standing in place show me a very low level, a very high level, and now a middle level. Good. Can you change to another level with your whole body and then extend a body part out into space in some direction? Ready? Go. Good, look at all of the different directions your body parts can go.**

Comment on the various levels and body parts that you see being used by the students. Repeat this activity by asking the students to jump or leap to a place in the room, stop, freeze into a shape at a low level, and stretch different body parts.

Part 4. Have the students explore the locomotor movement of walking in different directions (forward, backward, sideward) and at different levels. A drum or music can be used to accompany this activity. Remind the students that they are using their own personal space in the room and to be careful not to invade the personal space of other students (do not bump anyone). Continue to follow the pattern of having the students stop when the drum stops. Repeat this activity, vary the tempo and the locomotor movements.

GATHERING ACTIVITY *(10-15 Minutes)*

The teacher may want to put peel-off sticker spots on the floor for this activity to help the students quickly find a spot on the floor. The stickers are placed on the floor in an arrangement that allows plenty of space around each spot. (This technique works especially well with young children.)

Part 1. The following instructions can be used:

Look at all of the spots on the floor. When I count to three, leap to a spot and make a shape in your personal space and freeze. Only one student can be on each spot, and please do not bump into anyone. Ready? One-two-three. Go.

The teacher should comment on how well everyone found a spot and what interesting shapes have been made. This activity can be repeated if the teacher chooses, or if the students had problems finding a spot without bumping into someone.

Part 2. The teacher can continue by telling the students the following:

Look down at your spot because this is your place for the rest of the lesson. Be sure you know where your spot is. Where is your spot? Is it near to or far away from the door? the windows? the chalkboard? a friend? How can you remember where your spot is? Let us practice and see.

I will beat the drum 10 times. (The beats will be regular and steady similar to a heart beat.) **You can use those ten counts to walk wherever you wish in the movement space, but you must be back on your spot by the count of ten—not before and not after. Ready? 1-2-3-4-5-6-7-8-9-10.** (The teacher should count the first few patterns to assist the students in knowing when to go and return to their spots.)

How many got back to your spot at the right time? Try our ten-count pattern again. This time when you get back to your spot, make a shape that pushes or stretches one body part in one direction. Ready? Go. 1-2-3-4-5-6-7-8-9-10. (The teacher should comment on the various shapes and levels the students have chosen, then have the students relax.)

What do you think will happen if you have five drum beats to leave and return to your spot? (Wait for a few ideas from the students.) Can you go as far into space as you could with ten counts? No, there are not as many counts which means that the time is shorter and you cannot go as far. You have five counts to go away from and return to your spot. Ready? Go. 1-2-3-4-5.

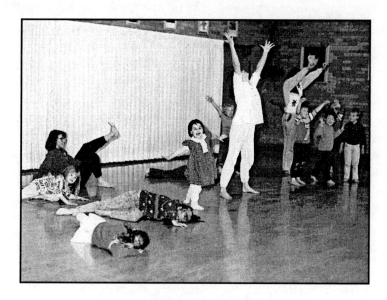

Branching Out

The teacher should comment on the success of the students with this set of counts. Repeat the 5-count pattern once more and add a "Branching Out" shape when the students return to their spots.

Part 3. The next part of the gathering activity increases the number of beats to fifteen for the students to leave and return to their spots. The teacher can provide the following instructions:

I will beat the drum fifteen counts this time. Will you have more or less time to get out into space and return to your spot? (Wait for an answer if possible.)

Yes. Good, you will have more time because you have more counts. Let us try. Ready? Go. 1-2-3-4-5-6-7-8-9-10-11-12-13-14-15. Many of you were able to go quite far and still get back to your spot by the count of 15. Very good. Let us try this again, but this time when you get back to your spot make a body shape that stretches out in space. Ready? Go.

1-2-3-4-5-6-7-8-9-10-11-12-13-14-15. Did you go way out in space and return to your spot at the right time? Were you happy with the shape you made this time? Well done. (Comment on the various shapes and levels the students chose.)

Part 4. Three patterns were introduced separately: a 10-count, a 5-count, and a 15-count. Have the students use each one of the three patterns consecutively. To complete the gathering activity, begin with the 5-count pattern; the 10-count pattern; and finish with the 15-count pattern. Ask the students to use a different locomotor movement to travel with each pattern, and to make a shape at the end of each pattern. Leave time between each pattern to comment on some of the shapes the students have created. Here is a suggested sequence.

1. Perform a 5-count pattern using **jumping** as the locomotor movement and making a shape that "branches out" in **one** direction after the students return to their spots.

2. Perform a 10-count pattern using **leaping** as the locomotor movement and making a shape branching out in **two** directions after the students return to their spots. (Two directions are used because this is the second pattern.)

3. Perform a 15-count pattern using **walking** as the locomotor movement and making a shape branching out in **three** directions after the students return to their spots. (Three directions are used for the third pattern.)

4. Repeat the above sequence and have students create shapes that "branch out" in their choice of direction(s). Remind the students that they can use various levels—high, medium, or low—when "branching out."

The underlying beat for all of these patterns has been a steady regular tempo. The teacher can add interest and challenge the students by varying the tempo of a pattern as well as the locomotor movements. The beats for a pattern can be very fast or very slow. Beats for a pattern could also be increased or decreased in tempo as the counts progress.

Remember that pathways (straight, curved, angular) and direction (forward, backward, sideward, diagonal) can be introduced as a challenging factor. For example, students could travel out in space using a forward direction and curving pathway and return to their spots traveling sideways in a straight or angular pathway. Again, the combinations of choices are many and varied.

RELAXATION (5 *Minutes*)

Have the students gently collapse on their spots and lie down on their backs on the floor. Ask them to take as much space in the position as they can with their bodies. They should stretch out as far as possible, then relax. Tell the students to sense how this "stretched-out" position feels— comfortable, uncomfortable, relaxed, tense, or some other feeling.

Have the students change their positions to become as thin, tight, and straight as possible. Tell the students to sense how this position feels— comfortable, uncomfortable, relaxed, tense, or some other feeling. Ask how this position feels in comparison to the "stretched-out" position.

Finally, have the students find a comfortable "space" or position and relax with the eyes closed. Breathe deeply and slowly a few times. Then have the students sit up slowly, and then stand. Use a locomotor movement and/or the counting that was involved in the lesson to take the student to their socks and shoes.

Outline of Lesson Plan One
"My Place in Space"

Unit title: *Space* Lesson title: *My Place in Space* Date:	Props/Materials: *Poem "Contrasts in Space"* Visual Aids: *LEAP* (diagram) *Diagram on board* *Spots on floor* Equipment: *Drum* Accompaniment: *Voice, percussion*
Objectives 1. *explore personal space* 2. *explore general space* 3. *explore directions & levels* 4. *Create a movement pattern*	

Activities of the Lesson	Formation	Time
WARM UPS 1. *Reach out all around - Poem - movement* 2. *Walk, leap - horizontal space* 3. *Jump - vertical space* 4. *Combination: Walk 8, leap 8, jump 4, rest 4*	*Circle:* *Sitting* *Standing* *Scattered*	*5 min.*
MOVEMENT EXPLORATION ACTIVITIES 1. *In place - how many directions can you reach* 2. *Shapes & directions in space* 3. *"Branching Out" & levels* 4. *Walking through space all directions & various levels*	*Circle* *Standing* *Scattered*	*5-7 min*
GATHERING ACTIVITY - *FIND YOUR SPOT* 1.) *10 counts - go away - return - make shape* 2.) *5 counts " " " " " "* 3.) *15 counts " " " " " "* *Combine above pattern & "branching out" shapes* 1.) *5 counts - jump - branch one direction* 2.) *10 counts leap - branch two directions* 3.) *15 counts walk - branch three directions*	*Scattered*	*10-15 min*
RELAXATION *Gently collapse on the spot* *Stretch out on back - Lots of space & make shapes:* *stretched out, thin, comfortable* *Relax and breathe*	*Scattered* *Lying on back*	*5 min.*
Evaluation of the lesson: 1. What went well? 2. What can be improved?		

OBJECTIVES

1. To explore levels of body movement—low, medium, high
2. To explore pathways—straight, curving, angular
3. To explore body shapes—straight, curved, angular
4. To create a movement pattern combining levels, pathways, shapes, and locomotor movement

WARM-UPS *(5 Minutes)*

Select warm-ups from previous lessons or Chapter 10. If possible, select activities that can be related to straight, curved, or angular shapes such as stretching, bending, twisting, turning, and swinging movements. Locomotor movements used could be sliding, galloping, walking, or another movement along straight, curved, or angular pathways.

MOVEMENT EXPLORATION ACTIVITIES *(5-7 Minutes)*

The teacher can introduce the pathways and body shapes by drawing straight, curved, and angular lines on the chalkboard as a visual aid for the students. The following instructions can be given:

We are going to explore how our bodies can move at different levels—low, medium, and high. We are also going to explore pathways of movement that take place in the air and on the floor (a floor pattern).

Let us begin by trying a body shape at a high level. Show me how high you can reach now. Can you reach higher? Good. Show me a shape at a middle level. Good. Now show me a shape at the lowest level you can reach. Good. Now stretch out on the floor on your back with your arms down to the sides and palms of your hands on the floor, legs are extended with ankles together.

While lying on your back lift your arms toward the ceiling by leading with the back of your hands. Allow your arms to continue until they are stretched out on the floor above your head. You have just made a pathway in the air with your arms. What

kind of pathway did you make? Was it curved, angular, or straight? (Accept the choices the students make.) **Let us repeat the pathway by raising your arms toward the ceiling (palms are leading) and bring them down to your sides. Good.**

Continue exploring air pathways for the legs. Ask the students to use different body parts to make air pathways that are straight, curved, and angular. Have the students change levels and explore movement sitting, kneeling, and standing. The teacher can select the levels or allow the students to make a choice of when to change levels.

Now explore floor patterns—pathways made by the feet on the floor as the students try various locomotor movements and become aware of pathways they select. Explore one locomotor movement and one pathway at a time, making sure that a variety of locomotor movements are chosen and that the three types of pathways are included. The teacher can use the following sequence for this movement exploration activity:

1. Have the students walk using (a) straight, (b) curved, and (c) angular pathways.

2. Have the students run using the three types of pathways. (Make sure no one bumps into anyone.) If the space is small, divide the students and have one group run at a time.

3. Have the students try other locomotor movements using the various pathways.

4. Create a locomotor pattern that combines two pathways. For example, skip in a curved pathway, then skip in a straight pathway.

5. Have the students create other combinations of locomotor movements and pathways on the floor.

GATHERING ACTIVITY *(10-15 Minutes)*

Combine pathways, shapes, and levels with a locomotor movement. Each pattern will include:

a locomotor movement traveling in a certain
        pathway (straight, curved, angular) and freeze in a
            shape (straight, curved, angular) at some
                level (high, medium, or low).

Three movement combinations have been created for the gathering activity. Accompaniment for this activity can be the teacher clapping or using a drum. If percussion instruments are available, however, the teacher could use one instrument for each combination—such as the drum for combination one, a gong for combination two, and rhythm sticks (or rattles or shakers) for combination three. Check to see what equipment is available in the school.

Another idea for accompaniment is to decide what instruments the students can make as a class project to contribute to this dance experience. The shapes and lines of the instruments can be related to the lesson: What shapes are the following instruments? Drum? (circular or round, or rectagular in the case of a slit drum), Claves or lummi sticks? (straight) A triangle? (angular)

The teacher can give the following instructions:

Let us make a movement pattern of pathways and body shapes. When I say "Go" run in a curved pathway without bumping into anyone. When I say "Freeze," you will show me a curved shape at a low level. Ready? Go. Freeze. (This will be Combination One: run, curved pathway, curved shape, low level.) (Repeat this combination.)

For the next combination, you will slide in a straight line (or pathway), and freeze in a straight, high shape. Ready? Go. Freeze. (This is Combination Two: slide, straight pathway, straight shape, high level.) (Repeat this combination.)

Our last pattern is walking in an angular pathway and freezing in an angular shape at a middle level. Ready? Go. Freeze. (This is Combination Three: walk, angular pathway, angular shape, middle level.) (Repeat this combination.)

Now have the students repeat each combination beginning with one through three. Then divide the class into the audience and the performers. Each group of performers will present combinations one through three twice to complete the gathering activity.

LESSON EXTENDERS

One way to extend this activity is to allow the students to individually select one locomotor movement, one pathway, one shape, and one level. The only accompaniment needed is for the teacher to say,

"Ready? Begin," and the students can use their own timing and direction for this combination. Students could use vocal sounds to accompany themselves and could make suggestions for the sounds that would work for a straight, curved, or angular shape or pathway?

Each student should hold his or her final shape and level until everyone is finished. Some students will finish earlier or later than others. Encourage students to complete their patterns and not hurry because everyone else has finished. This activity makes an interesting movement composition. The "show and share" could be used to allow students to see the variety of choices made for this movement pattern.

Another way to extend this lesson could be by recombining the pathways and/or shapes, and/or levels, and/or locomotor movement with each one of the patterns presented in this lesson.

Caution: This is a very complex lesson. Teachers may want to use just one combination as a gathering activity for this lesson, and then create three more lessons. Lesson two could incorporate the second combination and add on the first combination. Lesson three could incorporate the third combination and add the other combinations. Lesson four could introduce the "lesson extender"—having the students create their own combinations—and combine it with the other three combinations for a "grande finale" of this unit on space.

RELAXATION (5 *Minutes)*

The teacher can have the students complete the gathering activity and move immediately into the relaxation part of the lesson by using the following directions:

From your frozen position slowly move your shape to the floor and sit down. Now those students who have been the audience can find your place and sit down.

Select relaxation activities from the previous lessons or Chapter 10 to complete this lesson. Teachers may now be ready to create their own relaxation activities to finish this lesson.

Outline of Lesson Plan Two
"Moving Through Space"

Unit title: *Space* **Lesson title:** *Moving Through Space* **Date:**	**Props/Materials:** **Visual Aids:** *Draw pathways on the board* S I Z
Objectives 1. *explore levels* 2. *explore pathways (curved, straight, angular)* 3. *explore shapes (curved, straight, angular)* 4. *create a movement pattern*	**Equipment:** *Cassette/CD player* **Accompaniment:** *music*

Activities of the Lesson	Formation	Time
WARM UPS *(Select from previous lessons or Ch. 10)* *Relate lesson to pathways + shapes. Example:* *Stretch – bend (angular, straight)* *Swinging (curved)* *Pathways: slide (straight), walk (angular), run (curved)*	*Circle:* *Sitting* *Standing* *Scattered*	*5 min.*
MOVEMENT EXPLORATION ACTIVITIES *Levels – low, medium, high – in place* *Pathways in air – arms, legs* *Pathways on floor – walking: straight* *curved* *angular* *Combine <u>one</u> locomotor movement with* *<u>two</u> pathways – Skip: curved, straight*	*Standing* *Lying on back* *Standing* *Scattered*	*5–7 min*
GATHERING ACTIVITY COMBINATIONS: <u>*Locomotor Movement*</u> <u>*Pathway*</u> <u>*Shape*</u> <u>*Level*</u> 1. *Run* *curved* *curved* *low* 2. *Slide* *straight* *straight* *high* 3. *Walk* *angular* *angular* *middle* *Show + Share*	*Scattered*	*10–15 min*
RELAXATION *Select from previous lessons or Ch. 10* *Create new activities*		*5 min*
Evaluation of the lesson: 1. What went well? 2. What can be improved?		

QUESTIONS TEACHERS CAN ASK
STUDENTS ABOUT SPACE

Riggs (1980) suggested the following questions that will assist the teacher in guiding movement exploration using the element of space:

How many ways can I use the space I move in?

Can I move through space taking up very little of it?

Can I get from where I am standing to the wall in a straight pathway? [curved pathway? zig-zag or angular pathway?]

How can I use a lot of space as I move?

How do swinging movements make me use space differently from walking movements? Or punching movements?

How high or far can I jump? (p. 10)

SPACE WORDS FOR MOVEMENT EXPLORATION

Seefeldt (1980) suggested the following words that indicate movement in space and direction and in form and shape. These words can be explored individually or in combinations.

Space and Direction

up-down	forward-backward-sideward
near-far	around-through-between
over-under	front-back-behind-beside
in-out	away from-close to
on-off	
above-below	
toward-away	
left-right	

Form and Shape

alike-different	straight-crooked
big-little-small	curved-circular
large-small	round-square
wide-narrow	long-short
high-low	fat-thin

Words suggesting spatial relationships provide other ideas for movement. Students can explore the following movements alone or with a partner or small group.

meeting	linking	beside
parting	splitting	passing

The following poem may provide words for an innovative way for students to explore space and types of movements that the body would make in outer space, free from gravity.

Walking in Space by Grace Nash (1972)

Unfasten your seat belt, let go of your past,
Climb out of your spacecraft and close down the hatch . . .

Walking in Space, a new thing to me,
As one foot I lift, the other hangs free,
Like riding a bicycle? no pedals to race,
No wheels and no bars, just treading in Space . . .
No traffic, no hurry, no possible race,
It's lovely to walk in BIG OUTER SPACE.

My arms float so freely, swimmingly light,
I feel like a feather, slowly in flight
And stepping in clouds, with one foot or two,
I can draw circles wherever I choose . . .
Are you ready? CLIMB OUT . . .
(Toward end of walk, give these instructions:)

Back to your Spacecraft—
And close down the hatch—
Back now . . . to . . . EARTH,
And "Splash Down " at last . . . (Gong) (p. 39)

by special permission of Grace C. Nash, author. From Verses and Movement, Grace Nash Publications, Scottsdale, Arizona 85252, U.S.A.

SUMMARY

The element of space was described in this chapter. Some of the terms discussed and explored in this chapter were personal space, general space, direction, level, range, and shape.

Lesson One, My Place In Space, contained activities directed toward students exploring personal and general space. The gathering activity used a place (or spot on the floor) as home base from which the students would leave and return. Certain numbers of counts determined how far in the movement space they could travel before returning to home base.

Lesson Two, Moving Through Space, explored body movement in levels, pathways, and shapes. This lesson concluded with movement combinations that used a locomotor movement traveling in a certain pathway and a body shape performed at a certain level.

Questions teachers can ask about space and space words for movement exploration were included along with The Idea Page at the end of this chapter.

THE IDEA PAGE

7

FORCE

INTRODUCTION

Force deals with how much energy one expends in relationship to the amount of time used when performing movements. This category of movement is often referred to as the qualities of movement which are concerned with HOW we move. Qualities of movement deal with both force and time and include the following:

Sustained movement	— movement in which the action is maintained for a long period of time. The release of energy (force) is steady and continuous.
Percussive movement	— movement with a great deal of energy (force) that is released in a short period of time. Movements are quick, sharp, forceful, and somewhat heavy.
Staccato movement	— movement in a disconnected, sharp, quick, light manner
Pendular movement	— swinging movement that passes through the lower half of an arc. The swing is forceful at the beginning, has an element of momentum, and a point of suspension at the end of the arc.

(*continued*)

Vibratory movement	— movement with a quivering or trembling motion
Collapse	— movement best described as caving in

Along with the movements described above, other terms such as **heavy** and *light*, **strong** and *weak*, and **tight** and *loose* are associated with force or lack of force in movement. This chapter contains two detailed lesson plans that focus on force in movement. The first lesson explores percussive movement or strong movements. The second lesson explores movements that are contrasting between tight and loose. The other elements of body, time, and space automatically become part of each lesson, but expenditure of energy used in certain types of movement is the main emphasis in this chapter.

LESSON ONE—FORCE THROUGH MOVEMENT

OBJECTIVES

1. To explore percussive movements (the most energy or force released in the shortest amount of time)
2. To create a movement pattern that incorporates percussive movements and locomotor movements
3. To use poetry as an accompaniment for movement
4. To guide students in creating a movement improvisation

WARM-UPS *(5 Minutes)*

Select and adapt the warm-ups from previous lessons or Chapter 10. Include both nonlocomotor and locomotor activities in this warm-up period.

MOVEMENT EXPLORATION ACTIVITIES *(5-7 Minutes)*

(Sitting in a circle) Have the students listen to music that is strong, sharp, and forceful. One suggestion for music is "In the Hall of the Mountain King" Op. 46/4 from the Peer Gynt Suite by Edvard Grieg. "Beethoven's Fifth" is another good selection, or the teacher can select other music that may be suitable. After listening to some music, the teacher can ask the students the following questions, allowing time for answers:

What words can you think of to describe this music?
Do you think the movements should be fast or slow? weak or strong? heavy or light?
Sitting in our circle, show me a movement that expresses a strong, sharp, forceful movement, when I say "Go." Ready? Go. (Use words that the students have contributed. Repeat this activity using various body parts while sitting.)
Now, stand in place and try a sharp, strong movement as fast as you can each time I beat the drum (or clap my hands). **Ready?**

Beat the drum once for one sharp, forceful movement and comment on the movements chosen by the students. Repeat the drum beat several times (allowing time between each beat) encouraging the students to use different body parts, different levels (high, medium, low) and different directions. You may want to suggest making a strong, sharp movement with the head, shoulders, hands, elbows, hips, stomach, knees, feet, or other body parts. To achieve an honest and unanticipated response of percussive movement, have the students turn away from the teacher so that they cannot see when the drum beat will occur, now beat the drum and allow students to respond in their own ways. To assist the students in further exploration, the teacher can say:

This time when I beat the drum, make a strong forceful movement in some direction: up to the ceiling, down to the floor, out to the side, over to the corner, or some other direction you can think of. Make sure you have space around you so no one gets bumped. Ready? (Beat the drum several times varying the time between the beats to keep this activity challenging and interesting.)

Now let us walk around in the room as the drum beats quietly. When you hear a loud beat from the drum, stop and show me a strong, sharp movement. The drum may beat loudly two or three times in a row, so be ready with two or three strong movements. (Beat quiet walking beats and then the loud beat or beats. Repeat this activity a few times varying the length of time for walking and making sharp movements.)

As another movement exploration activity, the teacher can give the following instructions:

Find your own place in the room and sit down to listen to a poem. As I
read the poem think about the strong movements you will want to make
when we move to this poem.

A Strong Dance

Swing your fist up toward the sky,
Swing it down and up, <u>do</u>-try,
Now the other, swing it, too,
Your feet can't wait, they're stepping, too.
Swinging fists, and prancing feet,
Dancing strong, you feel complete—
When suddenly - - -
　　　You freeze into a statue! (p. 16)

by special permission of Grace C. Nash, author. From
Verses and Movement, Grace Nash Publications,
Scottsdale, Arizona 85252, U.S.A.

This poem can be repeated at least twice for the students to create their
movement patterns.

GATHERING ACTIVITY (10-15 Minutes)

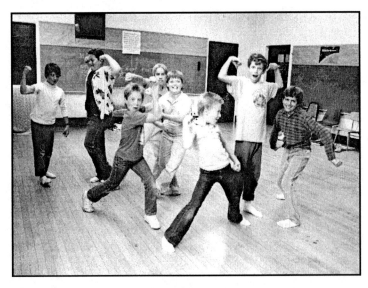

A Strong Dance

Using the music played earlier in the lesson ("In the Hall of the Mountain King"), ask the students to interpret the music using any locomotor movements they choose. Have the students stop to make sharp, forceful movements when they hear strong sounds from the music. Then have the students repeat their movement patterns.

Encourage the students to include any of the movements they may have explored during the reading of the poem, "A Strong Dance." The students should be able to travel in any direction and make sharp, forceful movements without touching anyone else.

Allowing the students to create spontaneously is called "movement improvisation." Improvising, or making up movements on the spur-of-the-moment, is a good way to challenge students. Movement improvisation allows the students to change any movements they wish, therefore, the first improvisation they perform will probably change as the activity proceeds. Observation of individual students as well as the group dynamics is also possible with a movement improvisation activity. The teacher will see interesting relationships occur among various students and the whole group while students are improvising. Students who feel shy about making up their own movements can be encouraged to copy a few movements of other students until ideas are formed.

Divide the group into performers and audience and have each group perform its improvisation for the other group. Play the music that has been used throughout this lesson. The teacher can instruct the students to begin when they hear the music, or any time thereafter, and freeze into a strong, sharp, forceful shape when the music stops, ending the improvisation. Repeat the performance with the first group of performers, and then have the second group of performers show its improvisations twice. Have the audience watch for the different movement patterns of the performing students. After the improvisation, ask the students questions about shapes, levels, pathways, and forceful movements. What did the students see that was interesting?

Time could be alloted in this lesson to show a videotape of the whole class improvising as well as the " show and share " groups performing. What did the students see that was interesting?

RELAXATION (5 *Minutes*)

Use slow quiet music to have the students stretch body parts as they are lying on their backs on the floor. Now the force used is very weak, light, and gentle. Repeat slow stretching movements in a sitting position. Have the students inhale in through the nose and exhale through the mouth, repeating this breathing slowly two or three times. (Select other relaxation activitives from those in previous lessons or in Chapter 10.)

Outline of Lesson Plan One
"Force Through Movement"

Unit title: *Force* Lesson title: *Force Through Movement* Date:	Props/Materials: *Poem "A Very Strong Dance"* Visual Aids:
Objectives 1. *explore percussive movements* 2. *improvise - movement pattern combinations* 3. *use poetry to accompany* 4. *students create improvisation*	Equipment: *Drum Cassette/CD player* Accompaniment: *voice percussion music "Mountain King"*

Activities of the Lesson	Formation	Time
WARM UPS *Select nonlocomotor + locomotor movements that relate to the lesson - see other lessons, Ch. 10, or create new activities*		*5 min.*
MOVEMENT EXPLORATION ACTIVITIES 1. *Listen to music "In the Hall of the Mountain King"* 2. *Describe feelings (strong, sharp, forceful)* 3. *Create movements* 4. *Repeat strong movements - various body parts, directions, shapes, levels, tempos* 5. *Poem "A Very Strong Dance" - create movements to poem*	*Circle or group sitting* *Standing Scattered*	*5 - 7 min.*
GATHERING ACTIVITY *Improvise movements using music + movement from above to create a piece (new movements can be added, too) Ideas for improvs: movements from warm ups, music + poem (movement exploration), and new movements Show + Share*	*Scattered*	*10 - 15 min.*
RELAXATION *Contrast - move from forceful or strong to gentle or weak* 1. *Listen to slow music, slowly stretch all body parts* 2. *Slow breathing*	*Circle or scattered Lying on back*	*5 min.*
Evaluation of the lesson: 1. What went well? 2. What can be improved?		

OBJECTIVES:

1. To explore tight movements (tension)
2. To explore loose movements (release)
3. To explore locomotor movements that use tight and loose movement concepts
4. To create a movement pattern

WARM-UPS *(5 Minutes)*

Select warm-ups from previous lessons or Chapter 10. Include some activities which use tight and loose movements, such as shaking body parts and then freezing the body parts. Also include one or two locomotor movements to get the students moving. Exploration of the concepts of "tight and loose" in relationship to locomotor movements is challenging. Questions such as the following can pose movement challenges: "Can you run (walk, leap, hop, jump, gallop, slide, skip) with a tight body? or a loose body? What locomotor movements seem loose or tight?"

MOVEMENT EXPLORATION ACTIVITIES *(5-7 Minutes)*

(Sitting in a circle) Use a piece of elastic or a large rubber band to demonstrate tight and loose. The following instructions are suggested:

What am I holding in my hands? Watch what it can do. (Stretch and release the elastic.) **The elastic can be very tight or very loose. What is happening to the elastic now?** (Stretch the elastic.) **Is it tight or loose?**

What is happening now? (Release the elastic.) **Is it tight or loose? Can you show me a body movement that is doing what the elastic is doing?** (Stretch the elastic.) **Look at all of the tight shapes. Can you show me a body movement that is doing what the elastic is doing now?** (Release the elastic.) **I see relaxed loose shapes.**

Let us try our tight and loose shapes again. Watch the elastic to see if it is tight or loose. (Repeat the stretching and releasing movements.) **How fast or slow does the elastic tighten or loosen? Watch the elastic first and then you make a movement that shows what the elastic did.**

The teacher should stretch the elastic slowly until it is tightly stretched, then release it fast. Stretch the elastic fast and release it slowly. Have the students stand and try this activity a few times varying the speed.

Now have the students explore tight and loose movements without the elastic-band demonstration. Encourage them to use different levels, different body parts, and different tempos. To help the students become aware of energy expenditure, the teacher can ask questions about how much energy or force is being used for tight or loose movements —a lot of energy or only a little energy? The teacher can then ask questions such as:

Can you try a tight movement with one arm? one leg? both arms? both legs? the middle of your body? or other body parts?
Can you make a tight movement with one body part and a loose movement with another body part?
How can you make some other tight shapes?
How can you make some other loose shapes?
Can you make a low, tight shape? a high, loose shape?

The teacher will be able to guide the students in creating many combinations of movements by choosing from levels, directions, tempo, and force (energy). Also the students should have the opportunity to create their own combinations involving tight and loose shapes and movements.

To conclude the movement exploration activity the teacher asks:

Do you think that you can make a tight shape and move around the room? Stay in your own space and show me a tight moving shape. (Students can select their own locomotor movements.) **Ready? Go.** (Allow time for exploring this combination.) **Freeze. Was this an easy movement combination? Why or why not?**

Let us make a loose shape and move around the room. Ready? Go. Freeze. Good. How did this movement combination feel different from the tight shape movement?

A movement exploration activity that teachers may want to try with the students for concepts of tight and loose is to ask questions about what "Things" are tight and loose. Tight objects could be shoes, clothes that pinch, or a space that is too small. Loose objects could be noodles or spaghetti, clothing, or "loose" change in a coin purse. What animals have tight and loose movements? A monkey might fit the loose category. A turtle in a shell might fit the tight category.

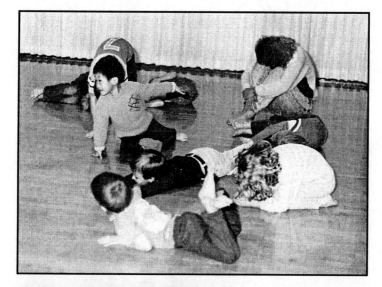

Tight Shapes

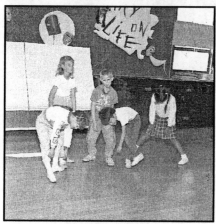

Loose Shapes

The students will contribute many ideas which can be used as movement experiments in exploring the concepts in this lesson. Asking questions about things that are tight and loose could be used as an introduction to this lesson, as an extension of this lesson, developed into the entire movement exploration activity for the 5-7 minutes within this lesson, or as a basis for a new lesson.

GATHERING ACTIVITY *(10-15 Minutes)*

To culminate this lesson the teacher can give the following directions:

Let us create a movement pattern that uses tight and loose and fast and slow movements. Show me a tight shape as fast as you can when I beat the drum. (Beat the drum and repeat the beat a few times leaving time between the beats for the students to make a shape.)

When I beat the gong, change your tight shape into a loose shape slowly.
(Beat the gong and repeat the beat a few times leaving time between the beats for the students to make a shape.)

Show me how you can move fast around the room in a tight shape. Ready? Go. (Beat the drum.) Freeze. Good. Can you move slowly around the room in a loose shape? Ready? Go. (Beat the gong.) Freeze. Good. (Repeat using a tight, slow movement and a loose, fast movement.)

Now let us create a tight and loose pattern. What shape should we make first? Tight or loose? How fast or slow should we make the shape? At what level should the beginning shape be? High, medium, low?

Let us try this shape now. Which locomotor movement should we choose? Walk, run, skip? How will our second shape be performed? Tight, loose? Which locomotor movement shall we use? What will our last shape and locomotor movement be? How tight or loose and fast or slow should it be?

The pattern will be a beginning shape (tight or loose), a locomotor movement, a second shape, another locomotor movement, and an ending shape.

Accompany the pattern with the drum and the gong (or other instruments that are available). The teacher can use 4 counts for the shape and 8 counts for the locomotor movements, or allow the students to decide how many counts for each part of the pattern. (There is nothing sacred about 4 or 8 counts!) Next try musical accompaniment. What sounds seem to indicate tight or loose? Would they be sounds that are high or low pitched, loud or soft, fast or slow? When the music plays, the students perform a locomotor movement; when the music stops, they make a shape that is tight or loose. This pattern (shape-movement-shape-movement-shape) can be repeated twice or three times in succession. If time permits divide the class into audience and performers for each group to see the patterns that the other students have created.

RELAXATION *(5 Minutes)*

The teacher can continue with the tight and loose concepts through the relaxation period. The following directions can be used:

Lie down on your back on the floor, legs are stretched long, ankles together and arms are down to the sides. Slowly raise the right leg up toward the ceiling and circle it, then gently allow the leg to collapse back to the floor. Repeat the sequence with the left leg. Repeat the sequence using the right arm and the left arm.

Close your eyes. Stretch your arms and legs out in any direction you choose. Keep stretching tightly, and then release or loosen the muscles of the arms and legs. Take a deep breath in through your nose and tighten your whole body. Very slowly let the air out through your mouth and let your whole body relax and become limp. (Give the students a moment of quiet time at this point.) Now sit up slowly, stretch, yawn, and stand up.

A Lesson Extender

To extend this lesson or create a new lesson based on the concepts of tight and loose, a circular elastic band can be given to each student as a prop. The students can explore tight and loose movements with these elastic bands. Musical accompaniment can continue as the students create their own patterns of shape-movement-shape. The students can decide the number of counts for the locomotor movement and the shape. The students can begin at the same time on a signal from the teacher. The second time this activity is repeated allow the students to begin when they choose. Also see Chapter 8 for props and ways to extend this lesson as well as other lessons.

Outline of Lesson Plan Two
"Tight and Loose"

Unit title: Force **Lesson title:** Tight and Loose **Date:**	**Props/Materials:** **Visual Aids:** Elastic
Objectives 1. Explore tight movements (tension) 2. explore loose movements (relaxed) 3. explore tight/loose combinations 4. create a new pattern	**Equipment:** Drum, Gong, cassette/CD player **Accompaniment:** Music, voice percussion

Activities of the Lesson	Formation	Time
WARM UPS Select nonlocomotor + locomotor movements from previous lessons, Ch. 10, or create new activities that relate to this lesson. Shake body parts (loose) Freeze (tight)		5 min.
MOVEMENT EXPLORATION ACTIVITIES 1. Use elastic to demonstrate tight + loose 2. Explore movement tempos (fast + slow) 3. Repeat tight/loose movements without demonstration 4. Explore tight/loose body parts 5. Locomotor movements - tight + loose	Circle Sitting Standing Scattered	5-7 min.
GATHERING ACTIVITY Class creates a pattern combine tight/loose - fast/slow. Choose: SHAPE, TEMPO, LEVEL, LOCOMOTOR MOVEMENT Beginning - (tight or loose shape) : SHAPE #1 Middle {locomotor movement = MOVEMENT {shape - tight or loose = SHAPE #2 {locomotor movement = MOVEMENT Ending (tight or loose shape) = SHAPE #3 show + share	Scattered	10-15 min.
RELAXATION (1) Leg lifts (tight), collapse gently (loose) (2) Stretch arms + legs + relax (3) Breathe in + tighten (inhale), Out-loosen (exhale) (4) Relax all body parts	Scattered Lying on back	5 min.
Evaluation of the lesson: 1. What went well? 2. What can be improved?		

QUESTIONS TEACHERS CAN ASK STUDENTS ABOUT FORCE AND FLOW

The following questions suggested by Riggs (1980) offer ways that teachers can guide students through movement experiences.

Force [Energy]
How loudly or softly can my feet touch the floor?
Can I make my whole body move strongly?
How can I move so I am as light as a feather?
Or as heavy as an elephant?
Can I move strongly then lightly using only my hands and arms?
Or just my feet and legs?
How hard can I push off the ground to get high in the air?

Flow [Bound, Balanced, Free]
What can I do that is easy to stop or "freeze"?
Can I spin around and stop quickly?
Can I roll more than once without stopping?
Can I jump and run and roll?
Or jump and roll and run?
How can I move so I can stop quickly and easily?
How can I move so it is hard to stop?

FORCE WORDS FOR MOVEMENT EXPLORATION

The following words can offer stimuli for movement exploration in force or energy.

tension	relaxation	sustained
suspension	vibratory	collapse
percussive	staccato	expansive
contract	strong	light
weak	heavy	explosive

Nash (1972) suggested exploring movement by using the following contrasts in space, time, and weight. Each line can be explored individually or the line can be compared or contrasted with another line or lines. The lines have been grouped, but teachers can change this grouping. As each line is considered, the teacher can think of such words as heavy, light, fast, slow, opening, closing, or other terms which might suggest movement. Also teacher and students might experiment with creating combinations or lines that incorporate locomotor movements.

Bear waking up at end of winter ....
Butterflies spreading their wings ....
Turtles pulling into their shells ....

Lightning Flashing, Streaking ....
Fog
Fast moving, slow moving clouds ....

Milkweed pods opening ....
Tulips opening, closing ....
Folding, opening chairs ....
Elbows, (opening, closing) ....
Hippopotamus, slowly (lying down to sleep, getting up) . . . (p. 39)

by special permission of Grace C. Nash, author. From
Verses and Movement, Grace Nash Publications,
Scottsdale, Arizona 852S2, U.S.A.

The following poem provides words that relate to force, flow, and weight, and could be used to explore movement.

Slow Motion In Weights

(Standing)
A heavy weight hangs on one foot,
Lift it slowly, high as you could—
Hold it poised—until this sound (gong or clap)
Then down it crashes to the ground!

Now the other, lift and poise—
Down so fast it makes a noise!

Can you walk with weights attached?
Ten great steps and not one fast?
One foot starts; takes all your strength,
Now the other drags at length.

Body bending, forward pull
That heavy load, each foot takes more,
Heaving shoulders, straining back,
Keep on going, don't come back.

(continued)

When you get there, loosen weight
Stretch yourself, relax and wait.

Now your arm is oh, so heavy,
Lift it slowly, keep it steady,
Hold that weight - don't let it fall—
Now it drops!—10 tons in all!

Try the other, do the same
Lift it slowly, -10-tons lame
Hold it there until you can't—
Drop it, like hot elephants!

(Utmost of Gravity)
Lean from the waist - as if there were boulders,
Of hundred pound weight attached to your shoulders.
Now from your head, from your arms, they are tugging
But you keep on pulling as onward you're chugging.

Heavy and sodden and weary you go
Back to your base through ten feet of snow.
When suddenly —————

(Weightlessness)
The snow is no more — you spring in the air!
No weight in your feet, no gravity there,
Your body is light as a feather can be,
And it swings light, sprightly, as tossed by the Sea. (p. 42)

by special permission of Grace C. Nash, author. From
Verses and Movement, Grace Nash Publications,
Scottsdale, Arizona 85252, U.S.A.

SUMMARY

Force (energy) is the element described in this chapter. Force deals with how much energy one uses in a certain amount of time to perform a movement. These actions are referred to as qualities of movement. The qualities of movement defined were sustained, percussive, staccato, pendular, vibratory, and collapse.

Lesson One, Force Through Movement, explored percussive movements which are strong, sharp, forceful, and quick. A great deal of force is used in a short amount of time when a percussive movement is performed. A movement improvisation activity accompanied by strong, forceful music was used as a gathering activity to conclude this lesson.

Lesson Two, Tight and Loose, provided experiences in movements expressing tension and release of body parts, shapes, and locomotor movements. An elastic band was used to demonstrate the concepts of tight and loose. The gathering activity suggested was to create a movement pattern based on shape-movement-shape. The activity presented the combining of tight or loose shapes with locomotor movements that could be performed with a tensed or relaxed body.

Questions teachers can ask students about force and flow and force words to use for movement exploration activities were included at the end of the chapter. The teacher is encouraged to use these resources to expand the sample lessons or to create new lessons. The Idea Page completes the chapter.

THE IDEA PAGE

Chapter 8

PROPS AND OTHER STIMULI TO USE IN CREATIVE MOVEMENT

INTRODUCTION

A common concern of teachers is where to find ideas for creative movement or creative dance. This chapter is intended to provide the teacher with useful, enjoyable, and exciting ideas about "topics for movement."

Props and other types of stimuli suggested in this chapter will assist the teacher in developing creative movement experiences, and enhance the chance for students to enjoy movement and create beautiful patterns as a result of using these "helpers." Props include objects that can be handled and manipulated by an individual or by a group. Bean bags, scarves, streamers, hula hoops, and elastic bands are examples of props that can be used to explore movement.

The senses of sight, touch, smell, taste, and hearing offer stimuli which can be a springboard for creative movement activities. Ideational and emotional stimuli also offer avenues for creative movement expression.

Written symbols and designs provide another route for developing creative movement. Two types of written symbols are included in this chapter along with ideas concerning how to incorporate them into movement activities.

PROPS

Props are an excellent way to introduce creative movement to students. Props include such equipment as scarves, streamers, elastic bands, or other objects that the students can manipulate either individually or as a group. By using props, students learn how to manipulate the prop and develop a movement relationship with it and to it. Props can assist in helping younger students understand the relationships between themselves, an object, and the space in which movement takes place.

Props are fun and effective to use in conjunction with movement for any age group and ability. Students can focus their attention on the prop and create marvelous movement patterns which might not occur as quickly as when students are simply using space.

Nearly anything can serve as a prop as long as the object is safely constructed, appropriately introduced, and carefully used by the students. The teacher should watch for potential safety hazards when students explore movement using any prop. Anticipate what problems might occur if a certain prop is used. Instructions in safely "operating" the prop should be given and followed by all of the students.

Many items can serve as props for exploring creative movement. Brooks (1978) suggested several that are included (among others) in the following list:

scarves	jump ropes	chinese ribbons
hula hoops	hand puppets	marionettes
balloons	bean bags	newspapers
floppy dolls	beach ball	fans
toys	masks	elastic bands

stretch fabric tubes 2 to 3 yards used individually by a student to explore movement inside the tube (See the directions for constructing stretch bags in this chapter.)

a very large stretch fabric tube to allow several students to crawl inside and make shapes (See directions for size later in this chapter.)

parachute (or large pieces of fabric sewn together that "float" well)

display cards with symbols, shapes, letters, or numbers, mounted pictures (cut from magazines)

assorted textures (bark, styrofoam packing material, velvet, fur, sandpaper)

large pieces of fabric of differing weights

simple machines (egg beater, pop-up toaster, popcorn popper, mechanical toys)

cardboard tube (from paper towels)

rubber balls (at least 12 inches in diameter)

crepe paper streamers (or cloth streamers or ribbons)

elastics (continuous elastic bands should be 2 to 3 yards and tied in a knot to make a circle)

Challenge the students to add to the above list with their own props. They will contribute many excellent ideas for props and ways to use them. Props can be used as a teaching tool or a visual aid by the teacher to assist students in understanding many movement concepts that deal with body,

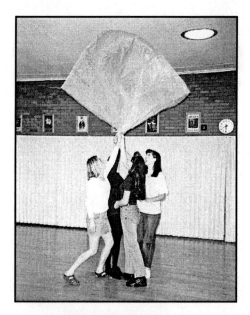

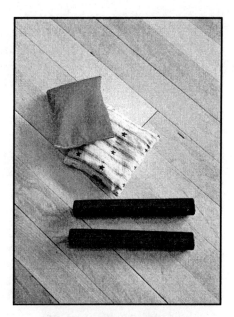

| "Parachute" Fabric that Floats Well | Bean Bags and Claves (Rhythm Sticks) |

time, space, and force. For example, an elastic band was used to demonstrate the concepts of tight and loose in Chapter 7, Lesson Two.

One prop for each student is important. Each student should be able to have his or her own prop when objects such as scarves, streamers, Chinese ribbons, elastic bands, bean bags, or hula hoops are used. Other props such as balls, dolls, parachutes, and fabric tubes can be shared by partners or by the whole class.

Each prop contains its own unique characteristics which should be capitalized upon when having the students explore movements with the prop. The format that can be followed for using many of the props listed is one of asking the students questions such as the following:

Is your prop heavy or light, tight or loose, long or short, small or big, round or square?

Can you make the prop move at a low level, medium level, and/or a high level?

Can you move the prop very fast, and very slowly?

Can you walk (run, hop, jump, leap, skip, slide, gallop) with your prop?

Can you do something with your prop while you are standing, sitting, kneeling, lying down, or balanced on one foot?

What other ways can you move your prop? or move with your prop?

These are only a few "starter" questions. The teacher will think of other questions as different props are introduced. Also, remember to ask the students to pose their own movement questions.

To guide the way for beginning to use props, ideas incorporating scarves, streamers, towels, elastic bands, bean bags, hula hoops, individual stretchy bags, and a large fabric tube have been presented below. Each prop carries with it some type of weight and force (or energy) required to manipulate the prop. Keep this in mind for helping the students to understand the concepts of body, time, space, and force.

Scarves

Scarves provide an innovative prop to assist students in creating movement. Learning how the scarf and the student move together can be explored by the teacher asking questions such as those previously suggested in this chapter. Scarves can be purchased at a thrift shop and laundered as necessary. If asked, parents would be willing to donate one or two scarves for your collection.

Each student can explore movement beginning with one scarf. For more interest and challenge, a second scarf can be given to each student with questions that help the students explore movement using both scarves in a variety of ways.

After exploring movement with the scarves individually, ask the students to find a partner and explore how two people (partners) and two scarves can create movement. Have each pair "show and share" while other couples watch and await their turns.

Musical accompaniment that offers a change in tempo and dynamics will help to stimulate movement exploration with the scarves. Music that incorporates fast and slow tempos and high and low sounds can offer an exciting challenge to the students. The best music that this author found for activity with scarves was the accompaniment for the dancing waters at Sea World in San Diego. The name of the album is Water Fantasy 2; the selection was "Salute to Rain" that provided slow and fast musical rhythms, including a tango to "The Rain in Spain!"

Another suggestion for accompaniment is music composed by Andreas Vollenweider. Additional ideas for accompaniment are discussed in Chapter 3. Also see other musical resources at the end of the book.

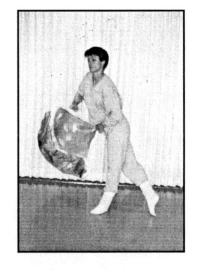

Movement with Scarves

Streamers

Use an approach similar to the one indicated for scarves, except substitute crepe paper streamers or long strips of fabric or ribbon (about 1/2 to 1 inch wide.) Crepe paper is fun, but can present a problem; young students may put the streamer in their mouths and the color tends to come off on the tongue and lips, but is usually not harmful.

Begin with one streamer and add other streamers as the lesson progresses, if this seems appropriate. For young students, one streamer may be enough to manipulate. The streamers should not be too long for very young dancers; watch for fatigue in the arms of the students, and finish this part of the lesson if the students appear to be getting tired.

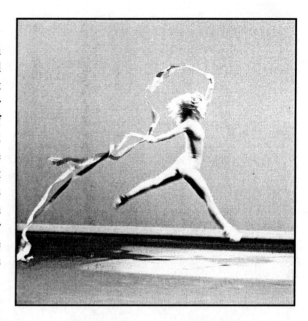

Movement with Streamers made of Ribbon

The same musical accompaniment used for the scarves can be used for streamers, or another type of accompaniment can be introduced. Scarves and streamers can be used to develop a lesson pertaining to sustained (steady and continuous) movement. By adapting the lesson on percussive movement ("Force Through Movement") that was discussed in Chapter 7, the teacher can substitute terms such as "floating," "on-going," "gentle," "easy," "gliding," and other terms that the students will suggest to build a lesson exploring sustained movements.

In an article, "Common Toys Make Uncommon Classes," Beech (1995) writes about several toys used as props for creative movement experiences including ribbon sticks. She makes her own ribbon sticks of:

> clear plastic balloon sticks (bought at a craft store for a nickel each); three-foot lengths of metallic curling ribbon in rainbow colors are tied to each stick ... These are favorites to draw circles in the air, wave about to music, or to hold while skipping and galloping (p. 78).

Towels

Bath towels or beach towels can be used as a prop to explore and understand weight and force. Texture, colors, designs, and shapes of towels can provide additional stimuli for creative movement exploration. Other ideas for movement with towels can come from the purposes for which towels are used such as: to wipe your body, dry your hands, put on your head after you have washed your hair, wipe up spills, or for suntanning. These ideas can be applied to ways a student can use the towel for movement/dance experiences.

Elastic Bands

A continuous circular elastic band can be made easily for each student. Measure the tallest student in the class from head to toe and double that measurement. The length of unstretched strips of elastic will be twice the height of the student. Cut the elastic and securely knot the two ends together to create the circular elastic band. Make one band for each student in class.

Make sure that the elastic will stretch easily to allow the students to hold the elastic under their feet and use their hands and arms to fully stretch the elastic above their heads. The width of the elastic is optional. A good width seems to be 1/2 - 1 inch. Lycra fabric (swim suit fabric) makes excellent stretchy bands that can be cut to any length and width desired. The teacher can have the students experiment with different widths of elastic and use whatever dimensions work the best. Elastic or lycra fabric can be purchased at any fabric store.

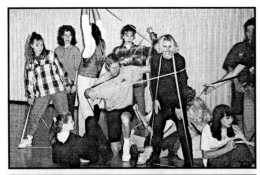

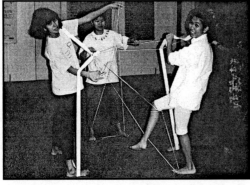

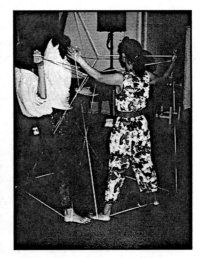

Shapes with Elastic Bands

With the students sitting in a circle, give each student an elastic band and ask him or her to begin exploring different shapes that can be made with the band while in a seated position. Refer to the questions in this chapter and at the end of Chapters 4 through 7 to guide the students in movement activities with their elastic bands. The teacher can also have the students:

1. Explore shapes with the elastic while they are: (a) lying down, (b) sitting, (c) kneeling, (d) standing, (e) using one leg and one arm, (f) using two legs and one elbow, (g) using the head, two arms and one knee. The activities can be performed using any level they choose. Teachers and students can create other combinations of shapes to try with elastic bands.

2. Walk with the elastic in some shape and move around the room (without bumping into anyone). The teacher can incorporate other locomotor movements for the students to try along with creating shapes with elastics.

3. Find a partner and explore the activities that could be tried with two students and two elastic bands. Increase this grouping to four students, to six students, and to eight students each with their own elastics combining all of the elastics to connect and create a complex pattern in each group. Have the groups explore ways to create one shape using all of the elastics, then explore different levels. Can the groups create moving parts or a moving shape?

4. Hold one very large circular elastic band and have the whole class explore movement and learn about cooperation. The elastic band can be in the center with the children on the outside of the circle, facing the center. Be careful when exploring movement that the students use equal "pull" on the elastic to begin the activity and then experiment with varying strengths of "pull" on the elastic by selected students.

The above ideas have been successfully used in the classroom. The teacher, however, will discover many other ways to use elastic bands as a way to help students expand their ranges of movement and thinking. Elastic bands can also be used to reinforce or extend Lesson Two—Tight and Loose in Chapter 7.

Bean Bags

Bean bags are an excellent prop that can be used to assist the students in developing awareness of body posture, balance, and hand-eye coordination. Bean bags are usually made of two squares of cloth sewn together on three sides into which dry beans, rice or lentils are placed and then the bag is sewn closed. Each student should have a bean bag for this activity. A good size for a bean bag measures about 4 inches by 5 inches.

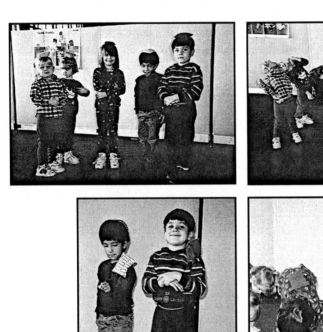

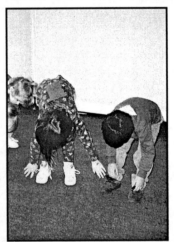

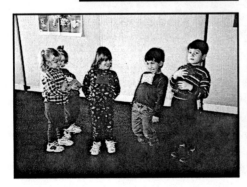

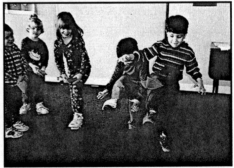

Bean Bags Explorations

The bag can be square, rectangular, triangular, or round in shape and can be larger in size if desired. Check the bags occasionally for splitting seams to avoid "spilling the beans!"

Students can learn to identify body parts by placing the bean bag on the shoulder, stomach, knee, elbow, back, and other body parts. Locomotor movements around the room will challenge the students to keep the bean bag balanced on a body part while moving. The teacher can name the body part (on which the bean bag is to be balanced) and a smooth locomotor movement like walking (which the student is to perform while keeping the bean bag balanced). Perfect accompaniment to begin exploring bean bags is a song entitled "The Beanbag" on a Hap Palmer Album, *Easy Does It!* (Order from Educational Activities, record number AR 581; see the address in the resource section.)

Tossing and catching a bean bag begins to develop hand-eye coordination and can be performed to music or a percussion instrument such as a drum. Musical accompaniment can aid students in tossing and catching their own bean bags. One suggestion is to select music that has a strong accent on the first beat of every measure and give the students movement tasks to perform when they hear the accent. They can toss and catch the bean bag when they hear the accentuated beat. Or the teacher can beat the drum, and each time the drum beats the students toss and catch their own bean bags. Also, the teacher can say "toss" and "catch" or simply allow students to toss and catch the bean bag without any accompaniment.

Various combinations of tossing the bean bag can be tried. The students can change hands or toss the bean bag back and forth from one hand to the other. The students can also work with partners and larger groups and play catch in various combinations (left hand to left hand, right to right, or left to right.)

Hula Hoops

[Created in 1949 by two Californians who observed Australian students in a gym class twirling bamboo hoops around their waists] Students can explore movement by using hula hoops (circular hoops of plastic) in various ways. Each student should have a hoop. One sequence for exploring movement using this prop is to have each student sit down in the middle of the hoop and place his or her hands on each side of the hoop and experiment with the ways the hoop can be used in a sitting position. Next, progress to a standing position, and then use locomotor movements in order to travel through space with the hoop. The use of such terms as "over," "under," "above," "through," "inside," "outside," and "around," can be used to help the students explore ways of moving in relationship to the hoop. The sequence in a nutshell is: (a) sit and explore, (b) stand and explore, and (c) locomote with the hoop. This activity can also extend to pairing and grouping to create movement patterns.

Encourage the students to add other descriptive words as they explore moving with the hula hoop. Also, challenge the students with the questions that were suggested earlier in this chapter. Other challenges can be offered by asking the students questions such as:

How many different shapes can you make while sitting inside your hoop?

How many different shapes can you make while standing outside of your hoop, but still touching your hoop in some way?

Can you hop around inside your hoop? Can you hop around the outside of your hoop?(Other locomotor movements can be substituted—walk, jump, or slide for example.)

Can you take two steps inside your hoop; two steps outside your hoop; then two steps inside your hoop?

How many different ways can you hold your hoop? With two hands? One hand, one foot, two feet, or other body parts?

Can you and a partner create a movement and a shape with your hoops?

The list of questions that can be asked is endless. Let the students select movements and ask questions of the class.

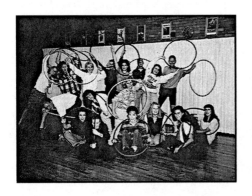 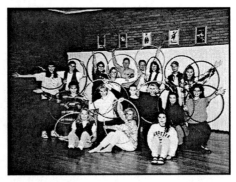

A "group hoop" Activity

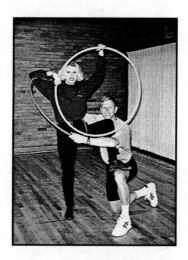
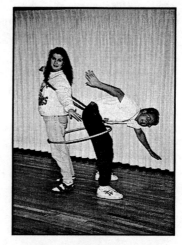

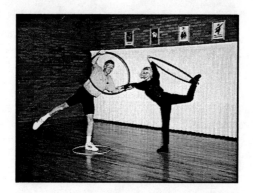

Partners Exploring Movement with Hoops as a Prop

Large Fabric Tube

A large fabric tube can be made out of stretchy fabric such as knits, stretch terry cloth, or lycra fabrics that have a two-way stretch (the fabric stretches in both the length and the width). The tube can measure about 5 yards long (or longer) and about 3 yards in circumference. The tube is made by sewing two *lengths* of the fabric together leaving both ends of the tube open.

The tube is placed on the floor and one student holds each end of the tube open for other students to crawl inside. These students can be called the "holders." About four students at one time can go inside the tube. These students can be called the "shapers." The "holders" squat down to the floor and close each end of the tube and continue to hold the tube ends closed on the floor as the "shapers" inside begin to create.

When the teacher gives a cue, the "shapers" will create a shape that changes the look of the tube. The teacher can use a verbal cue of: "high shape," "low shape," "wide shape," "a jagged shape," "any shape you want," or whatever the teacher wants to explore. The audience can make suggestions for shapes also. A drum can be used as a cue, so that each time the drum beats each "shaper" makes his or her own shape. Music can also be used and the "shapers"can interpret the music by making shapes of their own choosing inside the tube. Words of caution include:

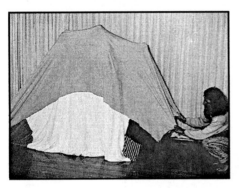 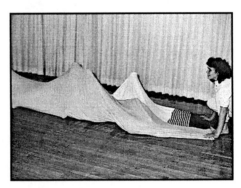

Shapers and Holders

1. Do not have the "shapers" inside the tube too long because the enclosure may frighten some of the younger students, and

2. Do not force any student to go inside the tube. Each student will try this activity when he or she is ready.

Repeat the activity by the "shapers and "holders" exchanging places. Then select a new group of "holders" and "shapers" making sure that everyone gets a turn.

A suggested sequence of activities for using the tube can be for each student to experience being a "shaper" at three different times. Each time, the teacher can use different cues for the group of "shapers." The beginning cue can be verbal instructions from the teacher as the students take turns as "shapers" and perform inside the tube. During the second round of this activity, the "shapers" will perform to percussion instruments and make a shape when they hear the instrument. For the third round, the teacher can select music that would permit the "shapers" to create movement inside the tube and interpret the music.

These three steps do not have to be used on the same day. Each round can be used as part of a lesson perhaps during the Gathering Activity. Explore the sequence and use what works best for the students and the time allowed for the lesson.

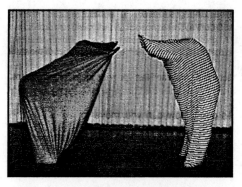

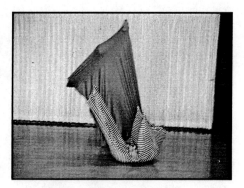

**Partners Exploring Movement
Inside Stretch Bags**

Bags: High and Low

Individual Stretch Bags

Select a two-way stretch fabric (stretch terry cloth was used for the bags in the pictures, other knit fabrics have also been used, and lycra swimsuit fabric is becoming popular). Measure the student from head to toe and double the measurement. Check the fabric to ascertain the direction of the greatest stretch and make sure that this goes around the body (horizontally). Cut two pieces of fabric to the approrpiate length. (Some fabrics are very wide; consequently, only one piece with the most stretch going around the body needs to be cut.)   Machine stitch the side(s) and one end of the bag using a zig-zag pattern. The "bottom" of the bag where the feet will be placed is stitched on each side about 1/4 the distance toward the center opening.   This technique provides a place for the feet at the outer bottom edges of the bag. Leave an opening in the center the for students to put the bags on over their heads, pull the bag down over their bodies, and put the feet into the spaces provided.

Cautions:

1.   Not all students will want to be enclosed in a bag. Those students who might feel frightened about putting the bag on and having their heads covered can put the bag on the opposite direction and leave their heads out.

2.   Before purchasing fabric for individual bags hold the fabric up to your eyes to see how much visibility is available for students to see. Attempt to select fabric that can be seen through when it is stretched. Some teachers have cut little holes for the eyes which is somewhat satisfactory in solving a vision problem. When students perform in their bags make sure that the space is safe from hazards such as chairs that might be bumped into and varying levels of the floor that could cause a fall.

OTHER STIMULI USEFUL IN CREATIVE MOVEMENT EXPERIENCES

Other types of stimuli can give ideas for movement exploration experiences. The senses, ideas, and emotions provide stimuli for movement.

Visual Stimuli

Pictures, linear design, color, and art forms provide stimuli for movement. Seeing a picture that suggests movement can help students learn to begin seeing the action, shapes, colors, and lines in the pictures. Since many of the lessons in this book focus on shape, the teacher can begin collecting pictures which have some basic geometric shapes. When showing pictures to the students, ask them if they can identify a circle, a square, a triangle, or some other geometric shape in some part of the picture.

Sign language used by the hearing impaired is also an excellent visual stimuli which provides students with a unique way to communicate. Signing is fun and challenging in learning the finger and hand gestures. These signs can be extended into large muscle movements to express a story, music, or other ideas that will be created. To begin such an activity, the teacher can invite an interpreter to present basic signs to the students and use this experience to provide stimuli to create movement patterns that incorporate signs. "Fundamental Dance Signs," a videotape created by Gallaudet University is a good video for ideas. To obtain this tape see the resources listed at the end of the book.

Additional ideas for movement can come from a picture as one looks for the geometric shapes, the lines (short, long, wide, or narrow), directions of the lines, colors, textures, and the subject of the picture. Students can create movements to express what they believe is happening in the picture. The students can be asked to bring a favorite picture to class and have the class create movements for this picture.

Tactile Stimuli

The sense of touch allows students to explore the textures, surface contours, shapes, and temperatures of props and costumes. Ask the students to close their eyes and be ready to touch something that the teacher will bring around to each student. Take a piece of coarse sandpaper, furry fabric, velvet, or some other object that has good texture, around the class to each one of the students. Each student will feel the object and keep secret what they think they have touched. When everyone has had a turn, all of the students can open their eyes and describe what they felt. The teacher can ask the students to move in a manner expressing how the object felt to them. The teacher can ask the following questions or make comments such as:

> Was it stickery, soft, smooth, sharp, fluffy, or (other adjectives that may describe the object)?
>
> How can you *move* in a stickery, soft, smooth, sharp, or fluffy way? Show me.
>
> If the object was cold with a curving surface, show me a movement that is cold and curvey.

The teacher will be able to think of many questions that will challenge the movement abilities of the students.

Olfactory and Gustatory Stimuli

The senses of smell and taste provide ideas for movement. Have the students use their imaginations to develop stimuli in this category. The teacher can say to the students:

> When something smells good, how can you move to show this?
>
> Show me how you can move when you taste something sour (or sweet, hot, or cold)?

Auditory Stimuli

Hearing provides the sounds of percussive instruments, musical instruments, the human voice, and verbal commands which give ideas for movement. The teacher can say:

> How can you move if the sound is soft or loud?
>
> Show me a way to move when you hear the tambourine shake.

Poetry and other words in Chapter 9 can be classified as auditory stimuli and can produce ideas for movement.

Ideational and Emotional Stimuli

Nature and the environment; moods and emotions; human relations; historical, legendary, or contemporary happenings; and literature can serve as stimuli for movement. Feelings provide a multitude of stimuli for movement. Entire movement activities can be created from emotions that we all share such as happy, sad, angry, frightened, or other emotional responses.

Colors

A combination of colors, emotions, and movement can become a creative movement topic. For example, the teacher can ask the students to express through movement how the color red (yellow, blue, green, or another color) makes them feel. An introduction to this activity can be a discussion about:

1.	Color of the object that is to be explored,
2.	The emotion expressed by the color,
3.	The speed this color makes the students want to move, and
4.	The force which should be used in expressing the color being explored.

For example, choose the color **red** and explore some of its details. Objects that are red include stop signs, apples, tail lights on a car, or fire engines. Red may stimulate emotions such as anger, fear, danger, or happiness (to many cultures), and may indicate a fast movement with great force. A pattern expressing the color red may include fast locomotor movements; strong, forceful shapes; and perhaps sudden stops depending on the choice of the students and teacher as they explore this idea for creative movement.

Multicultural Ideas

Multicultural connections can provide excellent stimuli. Movement can interpret events that are happening in society. One example is Kalediscope (a childrens' dance company in Seattle, Washington directed by Anne Green Gilbert) which created a dance expressing concern over the South African policy of apartheid. Children ages 8-18 were involved in creating this piece. Also many legendary characters, rituals, ceremonies, and events exist in every culture that can provide a wealth of material for creating dances.

Stories in literature provide many ideas that can be expressed through movement. Malaysian dance-dramas, Greek myths, Native American stories, and folk tales from around the world, provide well-known stories that have been passed from one generation to the next. Students can create their own movement-drama based on a story of their choosing. The teacher acts as a guide to help students explore all facets of the story and to select movements that express the theme. (See Chapter 11 for more ideas about creating dances related to cultural activities.) Childrens literature offers a feast of ideas about which to dance. Numerous books now comprise beautiful illustrations that can serve as stimulu for creating dances.

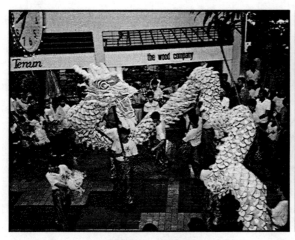

A Dragon Dance

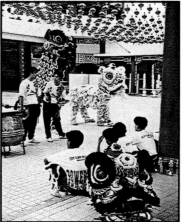

A Lion Dance

POETRY AND PROPS

The following poetry can be used with props or can be used alone to stimulate the students *to pretend* that they can move *like* a balloon or a scarf. Encourage the students to *feel* the dance rather than imitate the "properties" of the prop or topic.

The Colored Scarf

You're a gaily colored scarf that the wind blows through
Traveling ever onward with the sky so blue,

Downward toward the ground,
Upward toward the sky,
Westward toward the sun,
And you really don't know why.
A frolicking, a-rolicking,
You go where e're you're blown,
Until a someone snatches you
And takes you right on home. (p. 34)

by special permission of Grace C. Nash, author. From Verses and Movement, Grace Nash Publications, Scottsdale, Arizona 85252, U.SA.

Scarf Dance

(As students close their eyes the teacher places a
colored scarf in the hands of each student.)

Tiptoe quickly, to a space
Kneel there down into your place
Close your eyes, and sway your head,
Round and down and out, I said—
Open your eyes and gaze around,
Head and scarf go swaying round,
As you rise, (and stretching out)
Go dancing off and round about

Until - - - you hear the glockenspiel (bell sound) (p. 34)

by special permission of Grace C. Nash, author. From
Verses and Movement, Grace Nash Publications,
Scottsdale, Arizona 85252, U.S.A.

Jean Warren (1984) created the following movement
activities—"Balloon Poppers" and "Blow, blow, blow your balloon."

Balloon Poppers

Have the children pretend to blow up enough balloons to fill the room.
Then the children each decide for themselves where to tape a long sharp
pin (make-believe, of course) on some part of their body—the knee, toe,
elbow, nose, or hip for example. Set the balloon poppers loose on the balloons. They'll have to reach very low to get all the balloons in the room, no
matter where their poppers are. Great exercise!

Blow, Blow, Blow Your Balloon

(Sing to the tune of "Row, Row, Row Your Boat.")

Grab, grab, grab a balloon
Give it a big blow,
The more you fill it up with air
The bigger it will grow.

Blow, blow, blow your balloon
Perhaps now you should stop;
For if you blow it up too much
It will surely pop! (p. 71)

ADD-ON MOVEMENT GAME

The add-on movement game consists of combining the eight movement-related parts listed below. Numerous combinations of movement can be created from the list and the assumption is made that movement exploration of all eight categories has already taken place. The categories are:

1. Nonlocomotor (bend, stretch, etc.)   _____(bend)_____

2. Locomotor (walk, run, skip, etc.)   _____(gallop)_____

3. Direction (forward, backward, etc.)   _____(forward)_____

4. Time (slow, medium, fast)   _____

5. Level (low, medium, high)   _____

6. Force (weak, medium, strong)   _____

7. Size (small, medium, large)   _____

8. Pathway (straight, curved, angular)   _____

The "add-on movement game" begins with selecting one movement from number one and performing that movement. Next, select one movement from number two and perform that movement. Add movement number one to movement number two and perform both movements. Select one directon from number three and add on movements one and two. The five remaining sections are added gradually until all eight parts are combined into a movement sequence. The teacher and/or students can make one choice from each part to be added. This activity can be performed individually or in small groups. In this game, the concept of shape-movement-shape can still apply even though shape is not one of the eight choices.

The Add-On Movement Game helps students learn and remember a sequence of movements and improve concentration. New ways to use the add-on movement game will be discovered by the students and the teacher together as they explore this activity.

A CHART TO DEVELOP CREATIVE MOVEMENT PATTERNS

In Chapter 2, a chart was described to address the questions of What? Where? With Whom or With What? and How? The chart is based on the theories of Rudolf Laban (1975). The teacher may wish to use this chart to answer questions for preparing a movement pattern, or the teacher may wish to draw the four boxes of the chart on a poster, the chalkboard, or an overhead transparency and gather suggestions from the students. In Figure 7 the chart is presented containing suggestions for four basic questions that should be answered.

A Chart to Develop Creative Movement Patterns

1. **What** (Body Awareness) Whole body Body shape Symmetry/Asymmetry	2. **Where** (Space Awareness) Place, Shape, Focus Direction, Pathway Level, Size, Range Floor/Air Pattern
3. **With Whom/What** (Awareness of Relationships) Individual Pairs Group (small/large) Objects Body parts (how they relate to one another)	4. **How** (Awareness of Time and Force) Time: sudden/sustained quick/slow Weight: light/heavy Flow: free/bound

Figure 7.

Figure 8 depicts the Chart for Creative Movement Patterns without the suggestions included. This is how the chart would appear when drawn on a poster, chalkboard, or an overhead transparency. The chart can be filled in by suggestions from the teacher and the students. For example, select **what** body part and/or shape and decide **where** it will move, **with whom or what** it will move, and **how** it will move. Perhaps the students will select the whole body in a curved shape (what), will move at a high level using a straight pathway (where), in pairs (with whom/what), using quick light movements (how).

A Sample Chart for the Teacher

WHAT (Red)	WHERE (Blue)
WITH WHOM/WHAT (Green)	HOW (Orange)

Figure 8.

The teacher may wish to use the suggested color as a way to explore and express each category on the visual aid. A red marker would be used to write the body part or shape, a blue marker to describe the spatial action, a green marker to write a relationship, and an orange marker to note the time and force to be used.

DANCE CARDS OF MANY COLORS

As a way of expanding the use of color, the teacher and students may want to create a set of cards in each color with a "describer" on each card. Red cards could be used for a body part or shape, blue cards for spatial action, a green card for relationships, and an orange card for time and force. Or time and force can be separated and different colors used for each category—orange for time and yellow for force.

A card could be selected from each category and a movement pattern created based on the "describer" listed on each card. For example, a red card might list "arm," a blue card—"curved pathway," a green card-"pairs (partners)," and an orange card—"quick/light." This sample pattern is interpreted as using one arm of each partner, moving in a curved pathway in a quick, light manner. A fifth set of cards of another color could be made with a different locomotor movement (or traveling action) on each card. If skipping was selected for the traveling action, then the partners could skip while performing the other movements; they could also skip using a curved pathway.

The teachers and students can create a wide variety of movement patterns with these "dance cards" which allow opportunities for the students to make many choices and create interesting and fascinating combinations.

SYMBOLS FOR CREATIVE MOVEMENT ACTIVITIES

Waterman (1936) and her students created symbols to illustrate the basic nonlocomotor (axial) and locomotor movements. Figure 9 represents the symbols for these two movement categories. One symbol represents one movement.

For example, Figure 9 shows three walks, six runs, six tip-toes, and the figure continues with three repetitions of locomotor movements. The arrows for the gallop, skip, and slide indicate the direction in which the movement is emphasized. The gallop emphasizes a downward accent, the skip emphasizes an upward motion, and the slide emphasizes a sideways motion. Remember one symbol represents one movement.

Symbols for Movement

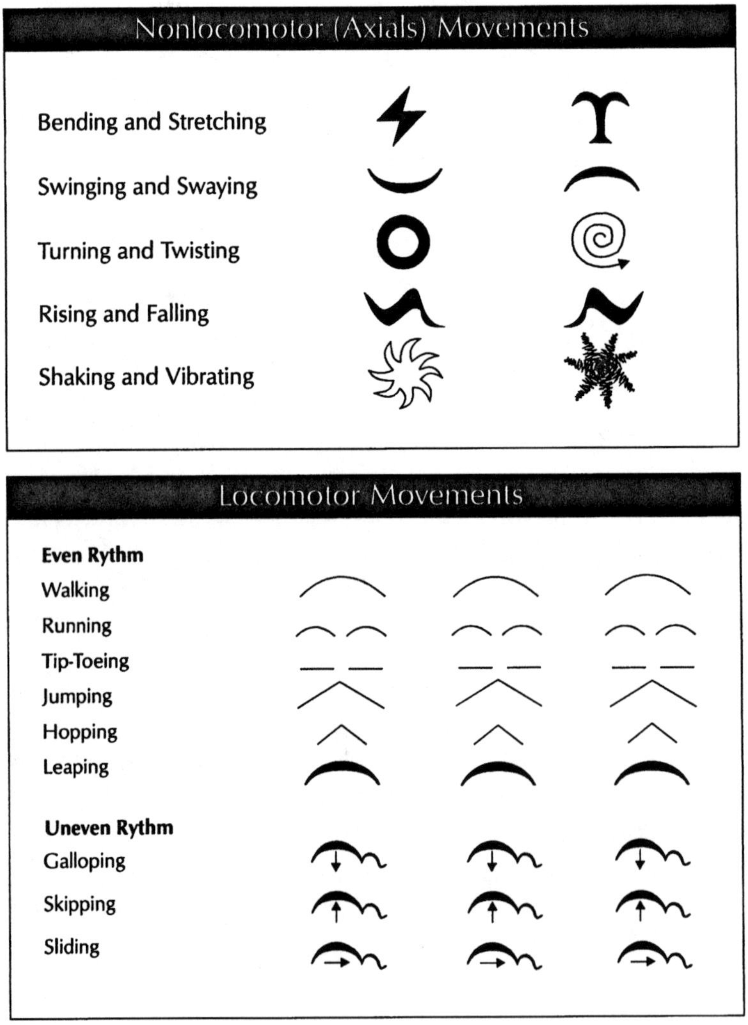

Figure 9.

The symbols use thin or thick lines. These line-width accents are perhaps more important when using the symbols in art projects to show an emphasis in the picture being created. When students are drawing these symbols, however, the emphasis does not need to be on line thickness as much as on understanding the symbol. For movement activity allow the students to draw the symbols as simply as they wish.

In movement, accents and emphases are seen when a mover makes changes in such aspects as: levels (low, medium, or high), time (fast, medium, or slow), force (strong or weak), or direction. Thick lines in a drawing could indicate heavy movements. Lines that appear high or low in the drawing could indicate a level change. One long continuous line may indicate a slow, sustained movement, while a series of dotted lines could suggest fast movements.

Waterman (1936) combined these symbols into movement patterns and also used them to create art projects or works of art. A picture composed of these symbols can be displayed on a bulletin board; this picture takes on a three dimensional form when movements are created and performed to interpret the pattern that was drawn on the paper. "Dancing your picture," could be the title of such a presentation. Sample "dancing pictures" are included in this chapter as examples of what students and teachers have created. One student even created a three-dimensional paper sculpture of the symbols selected for the movement pattern.

The use of symbols to depict creative movement will be discussed first followed by the use of symbols as tangible works of art.

Symbols to Depict Creative Movement

When written, the symbols developed by Waterman (1936) depict a "floor pattern." A floor pattern is a pattern that is created by the feet traveling around the room but is invisible on the floor surface. If we walked on the beach, our footprints in the sand would make a "floor pattern." If paint were on the bottom of our shoes and we walked around the room, we would leave footprints that would create some type of floor pattern or design. (The concept of a floor pattern was discussed and used as part of Lesson Two, Chapter 6.)

The pilot project (mentioned in Chapter 1) was one example that showed that developing a creative movement lesson based on these symbols was successful with children as young as preschool age. First, the teachers drew their own floor patterns based on the symbols from the movement chart. Their assignment was to select three nonlocomotor movements and three locomotor movements from Figure 9 and combine these movements in any way they wished. Each teacher showed the floor pattern she had drawn and then demonstrated this movement pattern to the class.

The teachers then took this experience to their preschool classes and recreated the symbols-for-movement process with their students. The best "recipe" for beginning was selecting one nonlocomotor and one locomotor movement and creating a written pattern followed by dancing the pattern. In one case the teacher and students even created a different set of symbols to use.

A sample floor pattern of one movement sequence is shown in Figure 10. This figure is included to illustrate a way to use these suggested symbols. Remember that the symbols developed by Waterman (1936) are only suggestions to assist the teacher in starting this creative art activity. The teacher and the students may want to develop some other symbols that are meaningful to them to express the basic fundamental movements.

A Sample Floor Pattern of One Movement Sequence

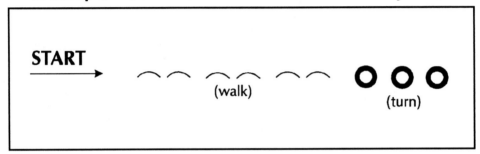

Figure 10.

An effective way to begin using written symbols as a stimulus for creative movement is to select one locomotor movement and one nonlocomotor movement, such as a walk and a turn. Decide how many times each movement will be performed. Let us say that a class has decided to take 6 walking steps forward and 3 turns. Figure 10 shows this pattern. The arrow in Figure 10 indicates the direction the dancer is moving. The arrow for the direction of the pathway does not need to be drawn, but using a symbol for starting and ending the pattern may be helpful.

Figure 11 illustrates how the pattern can continue by repeating the movement sequence. The change in direction of the second movement phrase, however, shows how the floor pattern and movement pattern can develop to use the available space and create a semicircular design. The words for the symbols are written in parentheses for instructional information for the teacher. In actual drawings, only the symbols should appear, as seen in Figure 12.

A Sample Floor Pattern of
One Movement Sequence Repeated

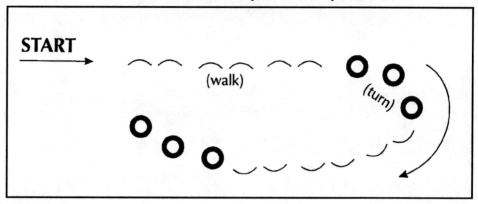

Figure 11.

Figure 12 illustrates a movement pattern that is based on the pattern in Figure 11. In between the two sequences, two nonlocomolor movements (one bend and one stretch) and one locomotor movement (4 gallops) have been added along with another curve in the pathway which increases the complexity of the written design as well as the movement pattern.

A Sample Floor Pattern of Increasing Complexity

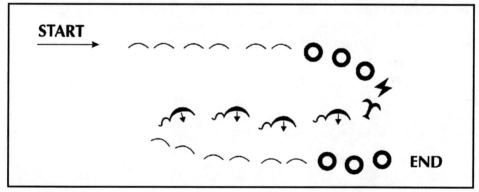

Figure 12.

Developing a floor pattern requires a number of decisions to be made which include:

1. Which movements will be selected from each category?

2. How many times will each movement be performed?

3. In what direction will the movements be performed?

4. How fast or slow will the movements be performed?

5. Will the movement pattern be performed alone or with a group?

6. If performed with a partner or a group, will the movement pattern be performed simultaneously?

7. Will the movement pattern be performed in the form of a "round" with groups or individuals entering at different times?

The tempo of the movements and amount of force (or energy) used in the pattern are not described by the symbols. Being aware of this factor, the teacher can help students incorporate time and force (energy) into the performance of their patterns. Another idea could be for the teacher and the students to create ways in which to express the tempo and the qualities of movement in the written design. The teacher can pose additional questions for student consideration such as:

1. How fast or slow will the pattern be? Which part will be fast, which part will be slow?

2. How much force or energy will be used in each part of the pattern? Is there a part that is very strong and forceful? A part that is sustained?

Symbols of Movement as Works of Art

Students love to draw and paint. All of their pictures incorporate some type of movement, shape, and line, even if the students are not attempting to draw specific symbols, such as those illustrated in Figures 11 and 12. Any drawings or paintings created by the students can be used as a stimulus for movement; consequently, begin examining the art work that the students create from the standpoint of translating their drawings and paintings into movement expression.

This activity can be developed into an extensive visual art project by the use of a variety of mediums to create the dance picture. Paint, pastels, crayons, colored pencils, or felt-tip markers, can be used initially. Texture can be added in the form of beans, seeds, rice, cake decorations, styrofoam "peanuts," and fabrics such as lace, rick-rack, ribbon, or other pieces of cloth. Glitter, metallic paper, or stars can add sparkle to the design. Teachers and students will be able to add to this list of materials that can be used to create these "dancing pictures."

The movement symbols presented in this chapter, however, can provide a good resource for a specific project. For a beginning experience, ask the students to select one movement symbol from each category (locomotor and nonlocomotor) and draw a picture. The symbols can be any size, any color or colors, and drawn any number of times the student wishes. Each student can share his or her picture and have classmates guess which symbols were chosen.

These symbols are like a language. If everyone uses the same symbols, reading another person's picture is possible; dancing your own or another person's picture is also possible. Reading and moving to someone's picture is challenging and fun. The teacher can assist the students in learning how to interpret the symbols.

One more addition to this drawing and movement interpretation project is the possibility of adding some type of accompaniment to the movements. Percussion instruments such as drums, gongs, rattles, rhythm sticks, vocal sounds, tambourines, and other instruments provide unlimited potential for interesting and exciting accompaniment for a group or individual presentation. Vocal sounds can make an interesting accompaniment. The student can begin by saying his or her pattern. In Figure 12 for example, the student can say one word for each movement (walk, walk, walk, walk, walk, walk; turn, turn, turn, etc.) or the student can say the name of each movement the first time it is performed and then contine to perform the movements as many times at the pattern requires. Music may provide accompaniment, but care must be taken that the music does not dictate the movement.

This project has great potential for programs where parents are invited to observe the accomplishments of their children. Parents will be able to see the pictures their children have created and then see these pictures brought to life through movement. Parents need to recognize and appreciate the importance and value that the arts bring into their lives, the lives of their children, and the life of the teacher.

The following designs, which were submitted by students and teachers, can be rotated and viewed either from a horizontal or vertical perspective. The emphasis of action changes with the rotation of each drawing. Try turning the pictures and observe the changing action and emphasis of each drawing.

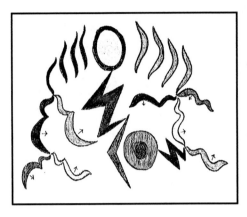 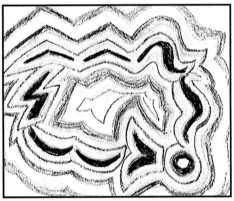

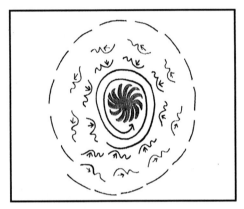 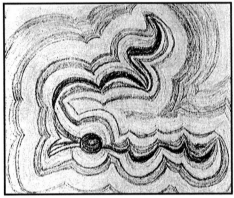

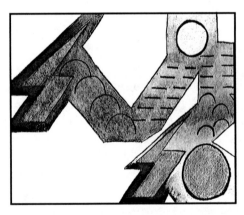 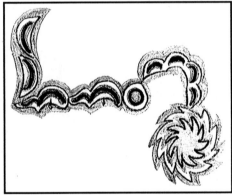

Movement Symbol Designs Created by Students and Teachers

(continued)

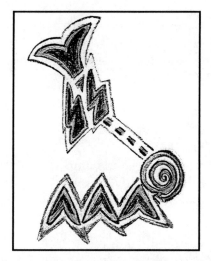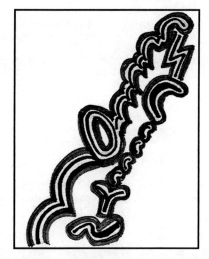

Movement Symbol Designs Created by Students and Teachers

GEOMETRIC SHAPES AND MOVEMENT

The following idea incorporates drawing geometric shapes, creating an animal or object for each shape, and designing a movement in that shape. Also another movement pattern can be created by using the types of movements employed by the animal that has been created from the geometric shape. Figure 13 shows examples of animals or objects created from a square, triangle, or circle.

Creating Animals and Objects From Geometric Shapes

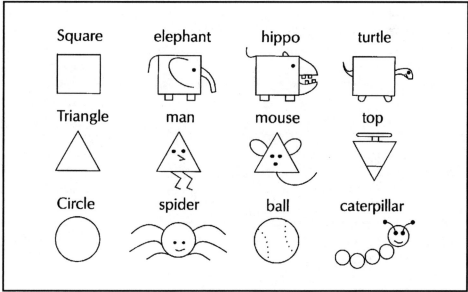

Figure 13.

Beginning with a square have the students make three animals and create:

> 1. A movement pattern expressing that shape and
>
> 2. A movement pattern expressing the types of movements made by the animal created.

Now have the older students choose one of the animals and divide themselves into groups according to the animal chosen. (For younger students, the teacher may keep everyone together and ask to children to select one animal.) Each group will then create a piece about that animal. For example, using the square in Figure 13 there would be an elephant group, a hippo group, and a turtle group.

Questions such as the following could be asked to help the students explore ways of preparing a movement activity:

> Is there anything alike/different about movements of these animals?
>
> Do they all like water? How do they move in water?
>
> How do they search for food? What do they eat, and how do they get it?

SUMMARY

This chapter discussed and gave examples of the use of props, stimuli, poetry, and written symbols that can be used in developing and exploring creative movement. The props included scarves, streamers, towels, elastic bands, bean bags, hula hoops, a large fabric tube, and individual stretch bags. The stimuli included those originating from the senses: visual, tactile, olfactory, gustatory, and auditory. Ideational and emotional stimuli were also discussed. Poetry for use with props or pretend props was included.

Charts, symbols, and diagrams for organizing and using creative movement were suggested, and the "Add-On Movement Game" was also introduced. Written symbols used to illustrate nonlocomotor and locomotor movements were presented both as an art activity and as a creative movement activity. These symbols can be presented by drawing the "picture" first and then using movement to interpret the picture.

Another written project of the geometric shapes of a square, triangle, and circle was presented. These shapes can be made into animals or objects, and a movement pattern can be created to express the shape and the movements that the animal or object would make.

New ideas that the teacher has learned from reading this chapter can be recorded on The Idea Page. Other ideas can be written on that page as they occur while teaching these lessons and through supplementary study.

THE IDEA PAGE

Chapter 9

NURSERY RHYMES, POEMS AND SONGS, AND WORDS

INTRODUCTION

Language, the written and the spoken word, contains rhythm and emotion that can be used as stimuli for creative movement activities. Words not only provide the impetus for creative movement, they also provide an excellent form of accompaniment for creative movement activities.

This chapter contains ways that nursery rhymes, poetry, words, and stories can be used to create or accompany movement activities. Nursery rhymes, poetry, and words can be incorporated into creative movement lessons during the warm ups, movement exploration, the gathering activity, or the relaxation time. Part of the creativity lies within the teacher's ability and imagination to explore and experiment with combining the spoken word and movement.

As soon as this chapter has been read, teachers can review the "words" at the end of the chapters for body, time, space, and force and use these words as a part of the lessons that they will create.

NURSERY RHYMES

Many nursery rhymes can be used to explore creative movement. The following list is one small sample of nursery rhymes that the teacher could use:

Jack and Jill	Pat-A-Cake
Jack Be Nimble	Little Boy Blue
London Bridge is Falling Down	Mary Had a Little Lamb
Row, Row, Row, Your Boat	Hey Diddle, Diddle

(*continued*)

Little Jack Horner   Pease Porridge Hot
Old Mother Hubbard   Hickory, Dickory, Dock
Little Miss Muffet

These nursery rhymes contain words and rhythm that easily lend themselves to movement. For example, "Jack and Jill went **up** the hill . . . Jack fell **down** . . Jill came **tumbling** after," provide obvious directional movements. The rhythmic pattern of "Jack and Jill" also suggests skipping, sliding, or galloping because of the uneven beat in the verse.

Jack be **nimble,** Jack be **quick,** Jack **jump** over the candlestick (suggests speed and action)

London Bridge (has a **falling** action)

Row, Row, Row, Your Boat (indicates swinging and circular movements)

Pat-a-Cake (calls for hand actions such as **clapping, patting, rolling** out the dough, and **throwing)**

"Pease Porridge Hot" [a thin pudding made of pease meal] can begin as a clapping game with partners. In a crossed-legged sitting position, the students sit facing each other and can say the verse and clap their thighs when they say "Pease," clap their own hands together when they say "porridge," and clap both hands with their partner's hands when they say "hot." Repeat the same sequence for "Pease porridge cold."

The last part of the verse, "Pease porridge in the pot, nine days old," consists of: clapping hands on thighs for "Pease," clapping their own hands together for "porridge," clapping the right hand with the partner's right hand for "in the," clapping their own hands together for "pot," clapping the left hand with the partner's left hand for "nine," clapping their own hands together for "days," and clapping both hands with the partner for "old."

You can remember the whole routine for "Pease Porridge Hot" by saying these cues:

Thighs, together, both (partners clap 4 hands together)

Thighs, together, both;

Thighs-together-right-together-left-together-both.

You have just clapped out "Pease porridge hot, Pease porridge cold, Pease porridge in the pot nine days old." Pre-school students may have a problem with right and left hands, but the teacher can adapt the activity by suggesting clapping one hand with your partner and omit the concern for laterality.

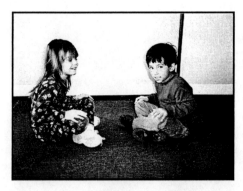

Pease   **Porridge**

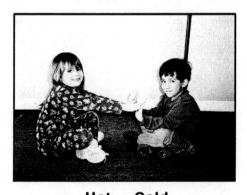   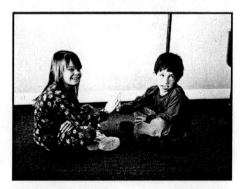

Hot   Cold   **(Pease porridge) "In the Pot"**

Pease Porridge Rhythm

A Sequence for Developing Nursery Rhymes into Movement

The following sequence of activities can be used with nursery rhymes, poetry, and dance steps. Weikert (1982) suggested that a four-step language process could bridge language and movement:

Step I	Say
Step II	Say and Do
Step III	Whisper and Do
Step IV	Do (Think and Do)
	(p. 16-17)

Based on the pattern that Weikert (1982) recommended, the following formula is suggested for exploring words and movement. A good formation for this period of exploration is to have the students and the teacher sitting in a circle.

1. Read the nursery rhyme (or poem) out loud to the students using an expressive voice (students listen).

2. Have the students say the rhyme with the teacher. One line at a time should be read by the teacher and repeated by the students. Finally, the whole rhyme should be repeated by everyone at the same time.

3. Clap out the rhythm of each line of the rhyme as it is spoken out loud (explore line-by-line and then the whole rhyme).

4. Clap out the rhythm of the rhyme as it is *whispered.*

5. Clap out the rhythm of the rhyme without speaking (but lips can move).

6. Together the students and the teacher create a locomotor pattern matching the rhythmic pattern that has been clapped in a sitting position.

7. In a standing position the students will move around the room performing the locomotor pattern that they practiced while sitting. The teacher can clap, use a drum, or say the rhyme for accompaniment.

8. Begin exploring the many possibilities of the movement pattern by:

   a. using different directions,
   b. using different levels,
   c. moving and saying the rhyme with no clapping, and
   d. using the locomotor pattern one time, stopping to perform a series of shapes during the second reading, and repeating the locomotor pattern once more.

Any part of the above may require repeating, especially if the students say "let's do that again," or if the teacher believes that repetition is necessary for further understanding. If music for the nursery rhyme exists, musical accompaniment can offer another variation. Music is available for many nursery rhymes including London Bridge; Row, Row, Row, Your Boat; and Jack and Jill. Music books for children and records, cassette tapes, or

CDs for children's music are available in most music stores or in the music section of major department stores.

Creating movements to some poetry may be explored best by the students on an individual basis; consequently, no need exists to create a pattern together and ask the class to perform the same movements. Also as the teacher and the students explore poetry and movement, the sequence of progression may be altered. Teachers should feel free to change any procedures or suggestions to fit their teaching styles and to meet the needs of their students.

This process of developing movement activities from nursery rhymes can be shortened as the students become acquainted with ways of exploring nursery rhymes, poetry, and words. The teacher will learn quickly how to bring these activities together for an effective lesson.

POEMS AND SONGS

Poetry and songs offer many opportunities to develop skills in creative movement. Many poems and songs possess movement words such as "jump, jump, went the little green frog," while others do not directly provide words for specific movements but convey a movement feeling.

Verses that contain action words provide an excellent and very clear way to begin working with words and movement. In beginning explorations, words and phrases can be used to guide choices of movements. As the teacher and the students become more skilled with creating movement to poetry, songs, nursery rhymes, words, and stories, however, expression and interpretation will become easier. The goal to reach as quickly as possible is for the movement to become less pantomimic and more flowing and filled with feeling.

Nash (1972) offered the teacher the following suggestions about how to use poetry in movement.

> The movement verses for the most part should be read with a rhythmical pulse that will encourage children to respond and move rhythmically.
>
> Rhythmical movement aids coordination and body control. Gradually as children lose their self-consciousness, there will come a flow of movement without the metered pulse which translates itself into a corresponding flow of speech, one complementing the other.
>
> When this improvisation in speech and movement occur[s], children will have attained a freedom in self-expressiveness that is admirable. And again, with encouragement they will create their own "poetry in movement," not necessarily in rhyming verses but more beautiful and refreshing than the metered or rhyming verse could ever be (p. 4).

A similar sequence of developing activities suggested for nursery rhymes is also recommended for poetry and song verses. An opportunity for the students to select their own movements to express the words should be built into the lesson, regardless of the source.

As soon as the verse has been explored fully, the teacher can ask the students:

> Are you satisfied with this particular movement?
> Have you thought about changing to another level?
> Does the speed of the movement seem appropriate?
> Can you think of other movements that you can use?

The poetry, nursery rhyme, or verses, can be repeated for another interpretation by the students, or each student can keep the movements already selected.

For a performance-and-audience experience to share the movement pieces, divide the class in half. The performers will find a starting place; the audience will sit down and show that they are ready by being quiet. The teacher will read the poem or verses for each performing group, and the audience will respond with applause when the performers have finished with a closing shape. The groups will exchange places, and the process will be repeated.

Libraries and bookstores should have a variety of poetry and nursery rhyme books available. The following list of poems and authors is only a brief sample of the selections that are appropriate for movement experiences and will likely be found in most poetry books for children:

"The Squirrel"	*by Christina Rossetti*
"The Spider"	*by David Barnes*
"The Eagle"	*by Lord Tennyson*
"Little Zobo Bird"	*by Frank A. Collymore*
"All the Fun"	*by Walter De La Mare*
"Fog"	*by Carl Sandburg*
"Choosing Shoes"	*by Frida Wolfe*
"Caterpillar"	*by Christina Rossetti*
"Shadow Dance"	*by Ivy O. Eastwich*
"Hands"	*by Dorothy Aldis*
"Feet"	*by Dorothy Aldis*

Folk songs and stories also provide students with an excellent lesson in the culture and customs of the country. The teacher can use the poetry sources available from the language and literature classes in the school and share them with the students and other teachers.

The best poets, however, may be the students in the classroom. Students can create wonderful poetry individually or as a group. With the teacher's guidance, the students' words can be stimuli for creative movement activities. Remember that poetry does not have to rhyme. It is a verbal expression about a feeling, thought, or idea. The teacher may want to have one lesson to develop rhyming words and another lesson to develop poetry that expresses feelings or ideas without rhyming qualities.

Additional Songs and Poems

The following materials include songs and poems that are ready for immediate use. All of the selections have been chosen because they have definite movement activities stated in the verses. The songs are sung to familiar tunes (listed in the parentheses) and piano music or recordings of the music should be available.

This book emphasizes the concept of allowing students to choose movements that will express their feelings; therefore, the students should have the opportunity to select many of the movements suggested by the songs and poems. The teacher's acceptance of the movements selected by the students is vital to the success of teaching and learning creative movement.

The following songs and poems are from English-speaking sources but the themes could be expanded to all cultural groups. The teacher can easily find other songs and poems from local resources that will provide material to enhance the movement skills of his or her developing students. Begin collecting other songs and poems now.

The following songs and poems were written by Jean Warren (1984)

Off We Go (Song)
(Sing to the tune of "Frere Jacques.")
Here's the train, here's the train
All aboard, all aboard
Chug-a-chug-a-choo-choo
Chug-a-chug-a-choo-choo
Off we go, off we go

Other verses:
Here's the airplane . . .
Chug-a-chug-a-zoom-zoom . . .

Here's the boat . . .
Chug-a-chug-a-toot-toot . . . (p. 79)

When Springtime Is Here (Song)

(Sing to the tune of "Here We Go 'Round the Mulberry Bush.")

This is the way we wake up and yawn
Wake up and yawn, wake up and yawn
This is the way we wake up and yawn
When springtime is here.

Other verses:
This is the way we sprout our roots . . .
This is the way we pop through the dirt . . .
This is the way we stretch and grow . . .
This is the way we shoot up so tall . . .
This is the way we open our buds . . .
This is the way we bend in the breeze . . .
This is the way we smile at the sun . . . (p. 45)

My Kite (Song)

(Sing to the tune of "The Farmer in the Dell.")

My kite is up so high,
My kite is up so high,
Oh my, just watch it fly!
My kite is up so high.

My kite is falling down,
My kite is falling down,
Oh no, it's near the ground!
My kite is falling down.

The wind has caught my kite,
The wind has caught my kite,
What fun, I'm on the run!
The wind has caught my kite.
(Repeat first verse) (p. 42)

Have You Seen My Feet? (Song)

(Sing to the tune of "Have You Seen the Muffin Man?")

Have you seen my dancing feet
My dancing feet, my dancing feet
Have you seen my dancing feet
As they dance on down the street?

(continued)

182 **Adventures in Creative Movement Activities**

Sometimes fast, sometimes slow
Sometimes high, sometimes low
Have you seen my dancing feet
As they dance on down the street?

Other verses:
Have you seen my running feet . . .
Have you seen my jumping feet . . .
(Substitute other movements the children want to
perform.) (p. 75)

Shadow Song (Song)
(Sing to the tune of "Skip to My Lou.")
Dance, dance, just like me
Dance, dance, just like me
Dance, dance, just like me
Little shadow, just like me.

Other verses:
Raise your hand, just like me . . .
Kick your foot, just like me . . .
Bend way down, just like me . . .
Flap your arms, just like me . . . (p. 36)

Little Shadow (Poem)
There is a little shadow
That dances on my wall
Sometimes it's big and scary
Sometimes it's very small.

Sometimes it's oh so quiet
And doesn't move at all
Then other times it chases me
Or bounces like a ball.

I'd love to meet that shadow
Who dances in the night
But it always runs away
When I turn off the light. (p. 36)

I See the Wind (Poem)
I see the wind when the leaves dance by;
I see the wind when the clothes hang dry;
I see the wind when the trees bend low;
I see the wind when the flags all blow.

I see the wind when the kites fly high;
I see the wind when the clouds float by;
I see the wind when it blows your hair;
I see the wind most everywhere! (p. 41)

Magic Feet (Poem)
One day I found a pair of shoes
Out upon the walk
They looked like any other shoes
Except this pair could talk!

They told me they were special shoes
That I might wear that day
I quickly slipped them on my feet
And headed out to play.

When I ran with all my friends
My shoes they went so fast
I found myself out in the lead
Instead of near the last.

And when we started jumping
Over brooks and streams
My feet just seemed to fly across
Like they do in dreams.

I wore my shoes in swimming
And swam across the lake
I looked just like a motor boat
And even left a wake.

Next I tried some dancing
The shoes were really neat
They let me spin and leap and bend
And never missed a beat.

(continued)

What a special day that was
What a special treat
To be the best at everything
To have two magic feet! (p. 74)

Wings of a Bird (Poem)
Flying fast, flying slow
Soaring high, swooping low
Swirling and twirling, and gliding through the air
The wings of a bird travel everywhere. (p. 55)

Four Little Birdies (Poem)
Four little birdies high in the tree
One flew away, then there were three.

Three little birdies with feathers so new
One flew away, then there were two.

Two little birdies out in the sun
One flew away, then there was one.

One little birdie alone in the nest
Afraid to fly out and join the rest.

Come little birdie, come fly like me
Come little birdie, fly out of the tree.

Flap your wings, flap your wings down
So you can fly over field and town.

Up, up and away the birdie did fly
Up over the trees, up into the sky.

Four little birdies now up so high
I almost forgot to wave them "Goodbye!" (p. 56)

Fleming (1976) included the following poem in her book. This poem is especially effective with preschool and primary age children during the winter season. Fill in the names of your own students when the appropriate part of the poem comes. This poem is a good relaxation activity.

Snowflakes

From behind a cloud one wintry day
Some little snowflakes came to play
They floated high, high up in the air
So high folks couldn't see them there.
They drifted contentedly round and round
'Til [_____] said, "Let's float on down."
So first came [_____] and then came [_____]
And [_____] and[_____], gently bobbing.
Then [_____] and [_____] and all the rest—
The snowflakes floated their very best
'Til gently and quietly on the ground
They finally settled without a sound.
And when folks pass them by they say,
"What a lovely snow we've had today." (p. 189)

One final poem in this section was written by Grace Nash (1972).

Seeds In The Ground

Curled in the ground so quiet and still,
Lies one tiny seed a-sleeping until
The sun and the rain with some kind of magic,
Reach down to the seed and whisper a secret.

Slowly it wakes and stretches one arm,
It stretches again, up through the ground.
Beautiful, - green, - a long slender stalk
Looks upward and nods to the one on the walk.

Out toward the sun three tiny buds come,
Unfolding, blossoming, a flower each one.
Beautiful colors that sway in the breeze,
Then finally they scatter their seeds, if you please.
(p. 35)

Suggestions by Nash:
Draw a pictures of the story; make a story ballet of the verse, with colored scarves for flowers.

by special permission of Grace C. Nash, author. From Verses and Movement, Grace Nash Publications, Scottsdale, Arizona 85252, U.S.A.

Dance in Poetry, edited by Alkis Raftis (1991), is an international anthology of poems on dance. Among the poets listed are: Emily Dickinson, Euripides, Thomas Hardy, John Masefield, Carl Sandburg, and William Butler Yeats. This collection of 118 poems about dance extends from ancient to modern times and is a wealth of material that provides a good resource concerning this area. The editor provided brief notes about each one of the poets.

STORIES

Many types of stories are available from children's literature as well as adult literature. *Ethnic Stories for Children to Dance* by Margery Dorian (1978) focused on the primary grades (1-4). Stories about America, Europe, Africa, and Asia along with stories for the holidays, and sections on rhythmic movement, music concepts, and dramatic concepts are included in this book. Although this book may be out of print now, a copy might be available at a library, a dance collection, through an interlibrary loan service, or from Dance Mart, an out-of-print dance books service (see the address in resources). Many books for children of all cultures are readily available from local libraries and provide wonderful ideas for telling stories through creative dance. Maurice Sendak's *Where the Wild Things Are* is a wonderful tale from which to create a dance story. The author's university student dance company created choreography that told Max's story and performed "Wild Things" for elementary school children. A few books are listed in the resources at the end of the book, and hopefully teachers and students will add to this list.

WORDS

A movement vocabulary and a speaking vocabulary develop in the same way. In language, we begin with one sound for speech and one letter for writing. Letters and sounds are combined to make words, and words are combined to make sentences. These sentences grow into paragraphs as the written and spoken languages develop.

A movement vocabulary is built in a way similar to a language vocabulary. One movement is explored and learned. Another movement is discovered and added to the first movement. Gradually a series of movements is created to express a feeling, an idea, or thought through a phrase. A series of movement phrases are "strung" together to create a dance. In language these would be paragraphs linked together to create a story. As the movement vocabulary develops, the student has a wider variety of choices from which to select exactly the right movements to express what he or she wants to "say" through movement.

Combining the verbal and motor vocabularies strengthens the student's abilities to develop a broad range of self expressive modes. One word can stimulate a movement. Boorman (1969) stated that when words expressing movement are linked together, a "sentence of action" evolves. She developed a selection of words divided into categories. Each word can be explored separately and then combined into sentences of action. The word lists appear first, followed by suggestions of ways to link words together to create a movement pattern.

As you read through the lists of action words, say the words aloud and consider the following:

1. How many syllables are in the word?
2. Is there an accent within the word?
3. What is the vocal tone (pitch of the voice—high/low)?
4. What is the duration of the word? (Is it spoken quickly, or can it be spoken for a long time?)

CATEGORIES FOR WORD ACTIONS

Percussive Actions
stamp
explode
patter
punch
pound

Traveling Actions

run	skip
creep	rush
flee	hop
slither	dart

Rising Actions
lift
rise

Sinking Actions
collapse
lower
fall
sink
drop

Jumping Actions

leap	toss
prance	soar
bound	hurl
bounce	fly

Vibratory Actions

shiver	shake
quiver	wobble
patter	tremble
vibrate	shudder

(continued)

Stopping Actions	Contracting Actions	
freeze	perch	shrink
anchor	settle	close
hold	grip	shrivel
pause		narrow

Expanding Actions	Turning Actions
grow	spin
release	twirl
spread	swivel
reach	whirl
open	whip

Other words can be added to the lists or new categories created as the teacher and the students explore words and movement, and then sentences of action. Boorman (1969) developed "sentences" of action which involve combining stillness (stopping) and action (starting) movements that were selected from various categories of action. (pp. 1-5) The following "sentences" are suggested as ways to begin.

```
patter-freeze
run-toss-grip
perch-twirl-gallop
tremble-freeze-dart-explode
explode-whirl-settle
```

If the teacher wishes to focus on jumping actions and traveling actions, words from those categories can be chosen, and a sentence of action can be built. The students may want to simply select several action words and not be concerned with the categories from which the words come.

Begin with a short one-line sentence. A second line can be added later to make a longer, more complex sentence of action. The sentences will naturally become more complex as the students develop skill in creating movement. As soon as the initial exploration of creating the sentence of action is completed, many variations exist to keep this movement activity creative and lively. Six variations are listed.

1. Use the same words in a different order:
   toss-perch-twirl-run
   run-toss-twirl-perch.

2. Reverse the order:
   whirl-freeze-flee-explode
   explode-flee-freeze-whirl.

3. Change the rhythm by repeating one word:
   toss, toss, toss-perch-twirl-run.

4. Change the rhythm by changing the timing from sudden to sustained.

5. Change the rhythm by changing the force from firm to fine (gentle) touch.

6. Change the rhythm by increasing or decreasing the size of action.

7. Change the articulation of the motion by emphasizing or using body parts.
   For example, perch can be explored on the feet, seat, shoulders, or knees. Twirl can be led with the head, palms of the hands, or an elbow.

Other Word Ideas

The following word groupings and listings are provided for further examination and exploration. These groupings include words which imply movement, movements in place, movements from place to place, gestures and pantomime, sounds, and group space words. A similar procedure can be applied to exploring these words and movements as was applied with the words in the sentences of action.

Mettler (1960) listed some words that *imply movement,* such as: search, hide, discover, hurry, meeting, greeting, parting, welcome, appear, and disappear; *movements in place,* such as wiggle, stretch, bend, twist, flop, drop, spring, bob, curl, lean, and jostle; and words that indicate *movement from place to place,* such as: crawl, creep, hobble, trudge, sprint, hop, leap, strut, and prance.

The following lists provide words related to gestures and pantomime, sounds, and group space.

Gestures and Pantomime

gather	mount	wallow	tug
skate	paw	pluck	grin
pump	wring	sweep	kick
freeze	fly	scowl	look
squat	inflate	hammer	run

Sounds

hum	sob	shout	gasp
talk	giggle	yawn	buzz
laugh	hiss	snore	sniff
chatter	roar	smack	

Group Space Words

collide	gather	arrange	weave
cuddle	expand	swarm	push
circle	squeeze	meet	bump
pull	hide	part	

The above words are in English, but the teacher can substitute or add the same or similar words in other languages for movement activities. Pairing words from different languages, in fact, is an excellent technique for combining movement and language arts development.

One of the author's all time favorite movement studies using words was created by university students in a modern dance class several years ago. Four students presented:

> "Plop, plop; Fizz, fizz;
> Oh, What a relief it is!"

This was a very popular Alkaseltzer commercial during the time. Other "fun" words that became part of a word movement study created by some other students involved "cottage cheese, cottage cheese; raisins, raisins, raisins!" which they said while they were skipping and jumping.

SUMMARY

Listings of nursery rhymes, poems and songs, and words that contain action were included in this chapter. Ideas for locating "danceable" stories were also included. Finally, ways in which to use these forms of words with creative movement were discussed. The Idea Page ends the chapter and provides a place for the teacher to write new ideas about words, songs, or rhymes.

THE IDEA PAGE

Chapter 10

ACTIVITIES FOR WARM-UPS AND RELAXATION

INTRODUCTION

This chapter is devoted to supplementary activities that can be used as warm-up and relaxation activities. Warm-up activities are presented first followed by relaxation activities. Additional warm-up and relaxation activities appear in Chapters 4 through 7.

WARM-UP ACTIVITIES

Follow-the-Leader Warm-Up

The teacher leads and the students follow the movements selected or created by the teacher. This is the teacher's chance to be creative, daring, spontaneous, and to have fun with the warm-ups he or she has chosen for the students to follow. Progress from floor activities such as lying down, to sitting and to kneeling, to standing in place, and to moving through space.

Begin with everyone sitting on the floor in a circle facing the center with enough space between each student to extend the arms and not touch anyone, legs extended, and hands in laps. Music of the teacher's choice can accompany the warm-ups, or the teacher can provide instruction throughout the warm-ups without musical accompaniment.

Nonlocomotor Movement Warm-Ups

Experiment with the following nonlocomotor activities:

1. Do a series of ankle flexions and extensions. (Flexing the ankle causes the soles of the feet to "look" across the circle to other feet soles. Extensions of the ankle can be thought of as pointing your toes.) The
(continued)

teacher can use terms such as "extend and flex," or "point and bend," or "stretch and bend." Use the terms that work best for the teacher and the students.

2.   Leave the toes pointed and extend the arms in front of the body, parallel to the legs. Flex and extend the wrists, then the elbows.

3.   Flex and extend the wrists and ankles simultaneously (both the wrists and ankles flex and extend). Switch the movements so that the wrists flex and the ankles extend, and repeat slowly several times. For a further challenge with this warm up, alternate wrist flexion and extension with ankle flexion and extension. (Right wrist flexes and left ankle extends; and repeat with the left wrist and right ankle flexing and extending.) Numerous combinations can be explored. The students will think of many combinations in case the teacher runs out of ideas! This same process can be used with knees and elbows flexing and extending.

4.   With the legs extended straight and toes pointed toward the center of the circle, let the fingers crawl down the legs and touch the toes, and crawl back up the legs, torso, shoulders, and reach directly above the head for a full stretch of the arms upward, and straightening of the back. Repeat this curling down to the toes, curling up, and stretching, several times. Varying the speed of this curling and stretching will keep the activity interesting. One time perform the sequence fast; another time perform the sequence very slowly. The teacher can also give directions, if necessary, otherwise the students can follow along by watching the teacher and being "copycats."

5.   From this seated position, the teacher can lead the students through bending, stretching, twisting, and turning at various levels—lying down, sitting with straight or bent legs, in a squatting or kneeling position, and in a standing position. Remember to do movements with as many different body parts as possible: head, eyes, face, mouth, neck, shoulders, arms, elbows, wrists, hands, fingers, legs, knees, ankles, feet, toes, and torso. The order of body parts chosen is selected by the teacher. Warming up with nonlocomotor movements at low to high levels prepares the students for locomotor movements that usually follow.

Locomotor Movement Warm-Ups

A good locomotor movement warm-up is to ask the students to walk (or run, skip, slide, gallop, or other movements the teacher wishes to develop) around the room to the beat of the music and when the music stops, freeze and make a shape. Repeat this activity several times guiding the students to explore high, medium, and low levels; directions of forward, backward, sideward; and the type of shapes they can make—wide, thin, twisted, round, or the teacher's choice of shape that may be part of the lesson for that day.

Balloon Warm-Up by Jean Warren (1984)

Let your children observe you blow up a real balloon. How does the balloon look before it's blown up? Afterward? What happens when you let the air out?

Have the children pretend to be limp balloons. As you pretend to blow them up, they expand, thrusting out their chests and opening their arms. After they have floated about lightly, let them pop each other with a finger so they deflate quickly. Deflating can be a little crazy with a large group. In this case, suggest that the children stand in a circle as they inflate so they can rush backwards without crashing into each other as they deflate. If the children have been holding their breaths as they inflate, the sound effects are great as they deflate (p. 70).

Wheels —Travel Warm-Up by Jean Warren (1984)

Pretend you are going on a trip. Begin on bicycles, showing the children how to lie on their backs and pedal with their legs. While you are pedaling, the children can decide exactly where they want to go.

Suddenly you hear a train. Now the children can hop aboard, making their arms move back and forth like wheels on a train. Hook together to form one long train by having the children line up and place their left hands on the shoulder of the person in front of them while continuing to rotate their right hands like train wheels.

When the children tire of the train, toot the whistle and call "All out for _____!" (wherever the students decided to go). For the return trip, recommend they take a plane to make the trip short. After they have zoomed around the room, their radar signals working to prevent any mid-air collisions, the children can circle the airfield, drop their landing gear, and take turns landing (p. 78).

Hints for Warm-Ups

1. Vary the speed of movements—some fast, some slow, some held for a good stretch, and other quick movements to change levels.

2. Use movements that are challenging but accessible to everyone's ability.

3. Include movements that require balancing on a body part occasionally. The V-seat is fun and challenging. It is performed while sitting on the floor. Sit with feet flat on the floor and knees bent, place hands on the floor beside hips with fingers pointing forward. Lift the feet off of the floor and straighten the knees keeping the legs together and toes pointed. The hips and hands maintain the balance point needed. Lift the hands off the floor and extend the arms forward—arms and legs are fully extended out in front of the body—and make a V-shape. Bend the knees and elbows and return to the starting position.

4. Ask for and accept suggestions for warm-up activities from the students and incorporate their ideas into the lessons.

RELAXATION ACTIVITIES

The following six ideas for relaxation activities are based on topics presented by Fleming (1976) in her chapter—Helping Children to Relax, (pp. 187-189).

1. **Clothes on the line.** Choose an article of clothing and pretend that you are hanging on the line with clothes pins holding you up. (Students could also pretend that they are folded over the line instead of being held up by clothes pins.)

   The wind begins to blow gently, then it blows more and more until the clothes pins are pulled off, one at a time. Suddenly one body part drops as the wind pulls the pin off, then another body part drops. As the wind keeps blowing all of the clothes pins pop off and the _ _ _ _ _ _ [article of clothing, shirt, sarong, blouse, or whatever the student has chosen] falls to the ground.

2. **Ice cream cones.** Pretend that you are an ice cream bar or ice cream cone in the hot sun. You begin to drip down your sides and melt. Slowly you melt down and grow smaller and smaller until you melt into a small spot on the ground.

   (continued)

3. **Kittens.** Do I see lots of tiny kittens curled up in little balls? I think I do! Let me look over here, I see some kittens opening their eyes, stretching one paw, then the other paw. All of the kittens are stretching all of their paws. Now the kittens have quietly curled up in a little ball and have gone back to sleep.

4. **Quiet music.** I like quiet music. I can close my eyes and think my own thoughts. Sometimes I like to move slowly and stretch to the quiet music. Other times I like to just lie still and let my arms and legs go limp as I listen to the quiet music. (Play some quiet music following these comments.)

5. **Sea gulls.** Pretend that you are a seagull and say: "I am a seagull, and I'm flying over the sea. I gently glide and softly swoop and sail and swoop right down to the sea" (p. 189).

6. **I am heavy, I am light.** "I am making my whole *self heavy*—I can feel heaviness in my feet, arms, back, and even in my tummy. No one could even pick me up. Now I am feeling *light, airy*, and soft as a breeze. I am letting go. My head feels as though it might just come off and blow away. I feel as though I don't even have a back bone. I am *so* limp and relaxed and light" (p. 189).

The following six "Relaxing exercises" are listed in Nash (1972):

1. Stretch to the rooftops and yawn if you can,
Let yourself slump, like an egg in the pan!

Now straighten up tall as stiff as a stick
Feel yourself tighten, let go with a prick!

Put out your arms and reach to the ocean,
Atlantic, Pacific without a commotion.
Bring your arms upward and touch at the top,
Then let yourself go, when you hear me say, "PLOP"

Circle one shoulder around and around,
Circle the other as loose as a clown.
Now circle them both and opposite go,
Like the Earth and the Moon in orbit, you know.

(*continued*)

2. Pull back your shoulders, bend elbows and place
    Your fingers on shoulders, like chicken wings laced.
    Elbows outstretched, Swing right one to front,
    As left one goes backwards, Keep swinging and jump:

    And-a-one, and-a-two, And-a-three, and-a four,
    And-a-five, and-a-six, And-a-now no more.
    Slump and relax, Breathe deep and exhale,
    Now you are ready for the next thing in store.

3. Dip your <u>hands</u> into a pail
    Shake them loose, to dry them well.
    Dip one elbow; get it wet,
    Shake it dry and let it set.
    Dip the other, deep down in;
    Shake it dry - and with a grin,
    Can you guess what next put in?

    Your <u>head</u> - that's what!
    please bend clear down - - -
    Circle it steady, roll it around —
    Slow to a stop. Reverse directions
    Until you <u>head</u> has <u>loose connections.</u>
    Now stand quite still and close your eyes,
    Compose yourself and breathe two sighs.
    Think quietly, relaxed and tall.—
    Open Eyes! - Blink fast - blink, blink—
    And that is all.

4. Bring your head down to your knees,
    Let your arms swing freely, please.
    Swinging, swinging, back and forth,
    Arms lead upward - soaring forth,
    Upward, upward, toward the sky,
    Drawing head and body nigh,
    Open hands and feel the rain—
    Now relax - - - Let's do again; *(Repeat)*
    [After the second time say] That's the end.

5. Pick out a place and kneel right down,
    Close now your eyelids and without a frown
    Let your head start to sway,
    Let it sway, where it may,

                                                (continued)

Let it sway, let it sway,
Let it sway many ways.
Now open your eyes,
And while you gaze around
Rise to your feet,
Pulsing head, shoulders, arms,
And dance through the room
Till the gong ends the charm.

6.   Move around as soft as fluff,
Till you hear the word, "Enough."
Now move around as hard as nails,
Firm as steel your body feels.
Once again so soft and light,
You move quite like a feather white.

Now stretch yourself like bands of rubber.
Taut and strained, walk to another.
Now let go, relax and feel
All floppy, flopping, not quite real—
Maybe you're a Raggedy Ann,
Or, A Raggedy Andy walking man.   (pp. 8-9)

by special permission of Grace C. Nash, Author.
From Verses and Movement. Grace Nash Publication
Scottsdale, Arizona 85252, U.S.A.

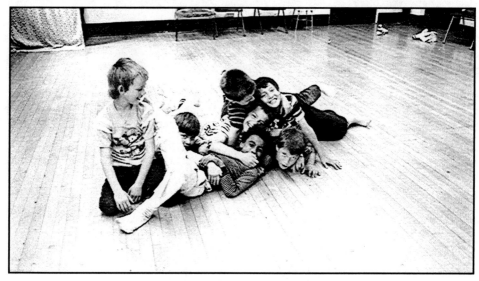

"And now . . . collapse"

SUMMARY

Supplementary activities to be used for warm-ups and relaxation activities were presented. The warm-ups and relaxation activities described in this chapter and Chapters 4 through 7 create numerous activities for the students. Students can also assist in creating warm-up and relaxation activities. The Idea Page concludes the chapter providing a place for the teacher to record new ideas about warm-ups and relaxation activities.

THE IDEA PAGE

Chapter 11

CREATING NEW FOLK DANCES
FOR
TODAY'S GENERATION

INTRODUCTION

Several years ago the author learned about a process for creating contemporary folk dances from a colleague, Theresa Purcell, an innovative professional who teaches dance and elementary physical education in New Jersey. The author assisted in piloting Purcell's ideas with children, university students, and classroom teachers in both Idaho and Malaysia. The dances created as a result of this process truly speak to the times in which the creators live.

Since beginning the implemention of this activity, an unbelievable number and variety of topics have surfaced about which the students choose to dance. Some of the topics have included:

Traditional Holidays	—	Christmas, Thanksgiving, Valentine's Day, St. Patrick's Day, and Easter
Personal Events	—	birthdays, graduation, and weddings
Sports Events	—	baseball and the world series, football and the super bowl, basketball, soccer, and hockey
World Events	—	the Gulf War and the fall of the Berlin Wall
Natural "Disasters"	—	tornadoes, earthquakes, floods, and volcanoes
Miscellaneous	—	"spud" harvest, hunting, parenting

The first time this author presented this assignment was to her university students in a Techniques of Dance class near the end of the semester early in the month of May. The students received Purcell's introductory information (to be presented later in this chapter) and their assignment for that day was to solve the problem of creating their own contemporary dance. Following a brief discussion, the group made its first decision of selecting a topic, which turned out to be Graduation Day since most of the students were graduating. They set to work creating their movement pattern, sequencing each part, and structuring their choreography to include a beginning, a middle, and an ending.

Here is their "dance blueprint":

1. Facing the mirrors (in the dance studio) in a line side-by-side, they donned their imaginary caps and gowns and made themselves look beautiful and handsome.

2. The procession commenced with the graduates following each other in a line that took a rectangular pathway and ended facing another part of the studio side-by-side.

3. Individually each dancer stepped forward to receive an imaginary diploma along with a handshake of congratulations, and stepped back in line to wait for each person to complete this ceremony.

4. Then a small circle was formed and a complete pattern of a Rumanian folk dance, Alunelul (which the students had learned the previous week), was performed.

5. The final gesture was throwing their caps in the air and heading for the graduation party.

The beginning — donning caps and gowns and preparing for the march and diploma ceremony

The middle — processional and receiving the diploma

The ending — circle dance of celebration and throwing caps into the air

The formula was to perform the dance twice; the first time without musical accompaniment, and the second time with music. Since this was the author's first attempt at teaching this activity, no idea existed concerning what topic might be selected. As soon as the topic was stated, however, the perfect music was miraculously located—Arthur Fiedler and the Boston Pops version of the "National Emblem March" which fit the movement pattern, gestures, and the theme so perfectly that an observer would have been convinced that the whole event had been pre-planned.

This was such an exciting experience to teach and share with the students that this creative dance adventure has been included in almost every one of the author's dance classes since then. This activity will work with nearly any age group from primary school through older adults; the youngest children taught by this author were first graders in Idaho Falls, Idaho who created a wonderful autumn dance.

Abundant thanks and grateful appreciation are extended to Theresa Purcell for granting permission to use information from two of her "handout" materials for creating contemporary folk dances. Her most recent model, "Creating New Folk Dances for Today's Generation (1995), is presented first, followed by an example of a dance using the theme of the "Birthday Celebration" dance that Purcell created in an earlier model, "Creating Contemporary Folk Dances" (about 1990).

THERESA PURCELL'S MODEL

Folk dances, traditional and contemporary, reflect the traditions, beliefs, and values of a culture. The dances communicate and express to the present and future generations the importance of recognizing and remembering significant events, places, and people of a specific culture. Dance symbolizes the great ecstasies and tragedies of the human race. In contemporary folk dance current events, customs, experiences and lifestyles are used as a resource for the creating [of] new folk dances. Every day newspaper headlines provide an account of what is happening in the United States and around the world. This written text reflects our contemporary society and becomes a record of the culture for future generations, in a similar way, dance also preserves the present day happenings and at the same time provides a means of expression of how we react, feel, and think about current issues, events and people. Through creating and learning dances we gain a deeper understanding and acceptance of the similarities and differences of the diverse cultures in our world.

Creating a new contemporary folk dance uses a process that includes: selection of a theme, development of the movement content, and designing the dance.

Selection of the Theme.

Contemporary folk dances reflect a theme that is relevant and of interest to the students. The dances can be based on current news events, a familiar custom such as shaking hands as a form of greeting another person, a personal event, occupations of the 1990's, or people in the news.

Examples of Themes.
Current news events
Space shuttle missions
Sports events
Weather related events - floods, eathquakes, hurricanes, drought
Freedom for a hostage
Takeover of a government
Inauguration of a new Governor

Personal events
Birthday celebration
Wedding celebration
Death of a friend or relative
Graduations ceremony
Family reunion
Holidays - religious or secular
Welcoming a new student to class
Celebrating a personal accomplishment
Winning a valuable prize
[Losing] a valued possession

Occupations of the 1990's
Teacher
Computer programmer
Astronaut
Surgeon
Fire Fighter
Artist
Bus Driver
Farmer
Telephone operator
Flight Attendant

Development of the Movement Content.
There are several approches to creating movement for the contemporary folk dance that express and communicate the selected theme. The teacher has the choice of creating the movement on [his or her] own or creating movement during the dance session with students.

One approach is to list the sequence of activities that describe an event. What happened first, next and how did the event conclude. Use simple phrases that describe actions. In a dance about a birthday celebration the sequence of activities can include, traveling to the birthday party, blowing out the candles, opening the gifts, playing a game, and going back home. Then movements are created to reflect how a person would move to illustrate the activity. Set the movements to a designated number of beats and practice performing the movement in unison as a group. Referring to the birthday celebration dance, the traveling movement may be on a bicycle. Students move their arms and legs and travel in a forward direction as if they are riding a bicycle. Added to the movement is a specific number of beats, sixteen forward in one direction then turn around and return to the starting place in sixteen beats.

Another approach to developing movement for the dance is to list words or short phrases that describe specific actions or emotions about the event, occupation, or person. Next create a traveling or stationary movement, or a still shape that reflects the meaning of the words. Movements can involve the whole body, or use only one body part. In a folk dance about the Midwest floods of 1993, six words or phrases describing the actions of the people or the water are listed, paddling, calling for help, building walls of sandbags, overflowing, receding and running swiftly. The words are translated into traveling movements and stationary movements. Each word or phrase is given a designated number of beats. Students practice the movements to the designated beats. To help create the movements, define the word or phrase using the elements of movement, body awareness, space awareness effort, and relationships. How will the action occur in space? What direction will the body move? Will the hands be an important body part in expressing the action? What type of force will be needed? Should the movements change levels or size? How fast or slow is the movement?

Designing the Dance.

Once the movement content has been developed, the sequence of movements and the spatial formation of the dance needs to be designed. Similar to traditional folk dance, contemporary folk dance is a communal dance. Dancers move in a common rhythm using the same movements. This uniformity of dancing brings the dancers together as a community expressing and communicating the same idea. The spatial formation can be a square, double circles, single circle, parallel lines or a single line. The formation can stay the same throughout the dance or change for different sections of the dance. Dancers can begin in a double circle, then form a single circle and return to the double circle for the end of the dance.

Choose a formation that represents the theme of the dance. In a dance about a birthday celebration a single circle is selected to represent a giant round cake. Another dance about occupations uses two parallel lines with dancers facing each other to represent a street with people living on two sides of the street. Circles are most commonly used in folk dance to represent a feeling of community, sharing, continuity, and the opportunity to see everyone throughout the dance.

The movement content for the dance is placed into a sequence. What movements are performed first, second, third. . . .? Folk dance movement is frequently designed to be balanced and symmetrical: moving forward then backward, to the right then left, one partner moves then the other; move together then apart. Movements are repeated and can occur in a pattern such as in the chorus-verse pattern or the ABA pattern used in music. Additional ideas for designing a spatial formation and sequence can be adapted from the spatial formations and sequence formats of traditional folk dances.

Author's Note: There are several compositional forms used to create dance choreography. Purcell (1995) suggested a common form of the ABA pattern. The following definition is presented to clarify any questions concerning this compositional form. Lockhart & Pease (1973) defined an AB and an ABA pattern as follows: An AB form is a two-part form "comparable to the verse and chorus of a folk song and typical of the structure of many folk dances." An ABA form is a three-part form and "is composed of an introductory theme (A), a contrasting theme (B), and a restatement of the original theme (A)" (pp. 84-85).

"The Birthday Celebration"

This dance was created by Purcell (about 1990) as an example of a contemporary folk dance:

Theme: A Birthday Celebration

1. Sequence of events: Traveling to the birthday party, blowing out the candles, unwrapping the gifts, traveling back home.

2. Dance movements: Students have explored the possible movements to express the events describing the birthday party and selected those movements they would like to use in the dance.

(continued)

3.   Dance design: This dance will use a single circle formation throughout the entire dance. Students begin facing the center of the circle. There will be four parts to the dance corresponding to the sequence that describe the events of the theme.

Part 1.   Traveling to the Party
Movement selected - riding a bicycle, the legs represent the pedaling motion and the arms moving from side to side represent the steering motion. The circle will move to the right first then to the left with students taking sixteen steps in each direction with the bicycle movement.

Part 2.   Blowing out the candles
Movement selected - Walking four steps up to the birthday cake, taking a four count inhale movement that bends the upper body backward, then exhaling to blow the candles out taking four counts as the upper body bends forward. Finish with four steps backward that will take the dancer back to [his or her] original place on the circle. The entire group of dancers will perform this movement toward and away from the center of the circle two times in succession.

Part 3.   Unwrapping the Gifts
Movement selected - Moving the arms quickly and at random in space while the legs are running in a small circle path using eight counts to complete the circle. This movement is performed to the right and then to the left. The design of this part of the dance is to have the dancers designated alternately around the circle as group A and group B. First the group A dancers will run around the group B dancers on their right, then repeat the run around the group B dancer[s] on their left. The group B dancers repeat the same movement to A on their right then A on their left. The stationary dancers can imagine they are the gift being unwrapped. They may want to move their [bodies] into a shape that would represent a gift.

Part 4.   Traveling back home.
Movement and design are the same as in Part 1.

In her 1995 "handout," Purcell added a part of playing a game at the party, and this could be used to extend the birthday celebration. Developing the playing-of-the-game part would be accomplished in the same way that the other parts of the dance have been created. Questions such as the following could be asked to help develop this part: What kind of game is being played? Are partners or a whole group playing? Is there one winner of the game or does everyone win? If there are prizes, what kind of prizes are they? Pin-the-Tail-on-the Donkey might be the game selected, then shaping this part would come as a result of selecting and creating movements for the various activities involved.

Many more themes can be added to the lists presented in this chapter; new categories can easily be developed as new folk dances are created. "The sky is the limit!"

SUMMARY

This chapter presented Purcell's (1990, 1995) models for creating new folk dances for today's generations. This author presented topics that her students have used to create contemporary folk dances, along with a description of "Graduation Day," which was developed by a dance techniques class. Purcell listed examples of themes such as personal events, news events, and occupations, as points of departure for (a) selection of the theme, (b) development of the movement content, and (c) designing the dance. Purcell's (1990) "A Birthday Celebration" was provided as a template for teachers to use in assisting students as they create their own new folk dances. The Idea Page ends the Chapter and can provide a diary of contemporary folk dance topics created by the students, or ideas for new dances yet to be created.

THE IDEA PAGE

Chapter 12

ASSESSMENT

AND

EVALUATION

INTRODUCTION

The 1990's have been years of increasing accountability on the part of artists and educators. Watchwords for this decade, like assessment, evaluation, outcome-based learning, expectations, standards, and achievement have become part of position statements such as The National Education Goals, Goals 2000, and The National Standards for Arts Education. Dance and the other arts have at least been recognized within the contexts of these various standards, and as a result may have the opportunity to "soar to new heights" in this new era of accountability— along with increased responsibility.

The apparent incoming tide of assessment and evaluation of students and teachers alike has demonstrated the need for a certain amount of coverage of these topics in this book. Therefore, in this chapter selected philosophical viewpoints about assessment and evaluation are presented, along with information about tools being designed that will assist in carefully measuring the progress of the teaching and learning process, especially as related to dance.

CHANGING ATTITUDES

The author's beliefs about assessment (the process of gathering information about student progress and teacher progress) and evaluation (the progress that has been made) have changed over the years. For example, in the "good old days" (in high school and college) we simply danced, created, and performed, and probably internally assessed our own achievements. That seemed to be good enough for that time, since no formal assessment techniques or instruments were readily available. Getting the dance finished was the true test of those times.

For approximately 35 years, this author has been teaching movement activity classes—swimming, rollerskating, bowling, archery, tennis, and dance. She has been teaching dance classes at the university level for 20 years; and every semester, finds herself wishing that she taught in the type of institution where no grades are required—the teacher is free to teach, students are free to study, all without the fetters of assessment and evaluation. The philosophy in this "ideal" institution would be that you teach what you teach, you learn what you learn, and you measure the achievements for yourself. Alas, most universities require a grade for each student, which includes the responsibility of creating a list of desired achievements or expectations which are ultimately measured in some way, and the student receives a grade according to achievement in comparison to the expected outcomes. At least in the university setting, assessment and evaluation are very important.

Along with teaching at the university, the author has also taught creative dance in preschools, kindergartens, and elementary schools on a continuous basis. Assessment and evaluation tools in these settings have been mainly observation, with some anecdotal records kept on a few "problem" children to chart their progress and demonstrate that dance makes a positive difference in their lives. No written examinations or grades have been given, the children are simply asked questions that will challenge their abilities to think, feel, remember, and create—their responses alone show to what extent they are able to perform these functions.

For two years, as a dance specialist at a child development center, individuals from special populations ranging in chronological ages from one year to twenty-four years old were taught. The assessments and evaluations were again conducted by observation and anecdotal records. The goal at the center was to hope that the students could remember some of the previous activity so that we could build on the next part of the dance. Again, the students showed that they remembered through their activities.

One of the major breakthroughs at the center was with a 12-year-old girl who spent the first several sessions screaming—unable to participate in any of the dance activities. The goal was to get her to dance more and scream less; one day this goal was reached—she danced and sang! The author's assessment of the girl was that she had finally "arrived." The journal evaluation was "we've made it!" She had passed the "test." No sophisticated quantitative measure was or really could be conducted, but she danced with no screaming—proof positive.

This experience was 20 years ago, and maybe times have changed. The "proof positive" of the child's observed activity still holds the teacher in good stead today in many settings, but can it "measure up" to the values of careful and caring assessment and evaluation of both students and teachers that are expected today?

Today, all teachers have the responsibility to develop skills in assessing and evaluating the growth and development of their students, not only for the sake of the increasing accountability that is being required in the 1990's, but for the sake of the students, to guide them sequentially along an appropriate "dance pathway." Dance, along with other art forms, has continued to struggle with credibility and recognition as a discipline; and the strides that have been made in the area of assessment and evaluation during the first half of the 1990's may help increase the respectability of dance and dance education in the eyes of our critics.

In preparing this chapter, the author's consciousness has been raised about (a) the philosophy of assessment and evaluation in dance, (b) the critical need for incorporating these processes into the dance curriculum at every level, and (c) innovative and appropriate tools that are being created by dance educators for this process.

ASSESSMENT IN DANCE EDUCATION

Assessment and evaluation of achievements within a discipline are vital to its growth and development. The only way to assure that goals and objectives are reached is to assess the outcomes and compare the results with the stated goals and objectives. Assessment offers validation for overall teaching and learning relationships. Over the years, authors of dance and physical education texts have increasingly addressed the topic of assessment and evaluation of student performances. These writers have provided a good basis for the future of dance assessment.

One group of authors, Hall, Sweeny, and Esser (1980), in *Physical Education in the Elementary School* included a very simple and effective tool to evaluate the progress of children in dance and rhythmic activities. They designed what amounts to be 4" x 6" cards that contain several aspects related to skill and attention when participating in dance and rhythmic activities. The evaluation form lists the area and skill being assessed and a box to check whether or not the student has appropriately completed the task. For example, in one evaluation tool, Hall, Sweeny, and Esser (1980) listed three *tasks* for the *skill* of rhythms identification in the *area* of rhythms and dance and asked that the teacher evaluate these tasks:

Clap to music
- —In rhythm
- —Not in rhythm

Walk to music as tempo is varied gradually
- —In rhythm
- —Can stay with tempo change
- —Unsure of rhythm, watching others

(continued)

Performance of the basic locomotor and nonlocomotor skills
—Adequate Skill Development
—High level of development,
—Problem area
[A space for additional comments is at the bottom of the evaluation tool] (p. 106)

Other evaluation "cards" presented have different areas, skills, and tasks that are assessed. The system appears to be simple, clear, and quickly accomplished in a positive manner. Unfortunately this book, which this author thinks is still one of the best texts for physical education and dance activities, is out of print but might be located in a university library. Also any library can conduct an interlibrary loan search. This book is worth seeing because it is simple, very easy to use, and includes good illustrations.

According to Mirus, White, and Bucek (1993):

There is a dearth of writing and research in the area of assessment of dance learning. Geraldine Van Gyn, commissioned by the Ministry of Education in British Columbia, Canada, to report on the status of dance assessment writes, "In an extensive search of the dance literature, only one article was found dealing directly with the topic of assessment and only three others dealt with the measurement of creativity as one aspect of dance product. While there are a number of sources which mention assessment, these sources describe only in general terms what may be assessed and occasionally a method of approaching the assessment." (p. 181) [Van Gyn and O'Neill conducted their research as recently as 1989.]

Several authors in the 1990's have addressed assessment and evaluation issues which respond to Van Gyn and O'Neill's concerns about the dearth of writing and research in the area of assessment of dance learning. Stinson (1991) presented a paper titled, "Promising Practices in Arts Education Assessment," and discussed some of her views about assessment, the Theory of Multiple Intelligences, and three kinds of artistic thinking which lead to her points about assessment at the preschool level. Stinson (1991) "hits the nail on the head" as she describes her feelings about assessment.

Assessment is one of the most troubling issues for all educators, one we cannot ignore in current times. It is particularly troubling for arts educators, who used to be able to ignore the issue, at least when dealing with young children . . . .

I must admit at the outset that I often find myself agreeing with Maxine Greene, who commented recently to me, "Why do we have to assess everything? Can't we just accept some things as important?" I think back to when my own children were young and we took trips to the zoo and other interesting places. My children and I were engaged together in something we each found interesting. I trusted that they learned during these experiences, but I felt no need to assess *what* or *how much* they learned. I *knew* it was a good way for us to spend the afternoon. I think the luxury of experiencing without assessing is still open to parents, but it is increasingly not open to teachers.

While I acknowledge the need for assessment in education, I am concerned about how we do it and what we use it for. Assessment is all too often used to categorize and rank children like appliances in the Sears catalogue, according to who is good, better, and best—and even who is not good at all. I mistrust quantitative and summative evaluation for this reason. It changes the way I choose to be with children, in which I value them as unique persons with their own qualities and abilities—and, yes, their own limitations—which make each of them wonderfully different from anyone else in the world. So when I speak of what I see as the most promising proposals for assessment, they are largely qualitative and formative in nature (p. 51).

Dance book authors such as Gilbert (1992), Purcell (1994), Wall and Murray (1994), Bennett and Riemer (1995), and Joyce (1994) have each addressed evaluation and assessment in various ways. In an adaptation of Van Gyn and O'Neill's 1989 fine arts assessment research, Gilbert (1992) made the following points concerning assessment:

Assessment in dance is essential if this art form is to become a basic part of public education. Learning occurs in dance and this learning can be assessed. Assessment provides information that is necessary if students are to continue to grow and develop. Assessment provides important information for the parents, the school and the community. Through assessment, students evaluate themselves, understanding what they know and what they need to know next.

(continued)

In order for assessment to occur, there must first be clear learning outcomes, curriculum goals and appropriate assessment tools which are tied to the outcomes and goals. . . . It is essential that all the learning outcomes (cognitive, affective, physical and social) be assessed. . . . Assessment tools can be designed in a variety of ways, when you have outcomes and goals firmly in place and the following ideas are taken into consideration.

Assessment is linked to the curriculum goals and reporting indicates the student's progress toward these goals, discussing both strengths and weaknesses, and includes suggestions for progressing further toward these goals.

Assessment is context dependent being specific to each student, taking into consideration [his or her] age, culture, and previous experience.

Assessment is carried out on a formative (process) and summative (product) basis with many indicators of progress being used such as anecdotal comments, journals, videos, checklists and tests.

Assessment consists of subjective evaluation based on objective criteria. The evaluator needs to have a good understanding of the learning outcomes (based on dance as an art form) in order for the assessment to be effective.

Assessment needs to be a collaborative and friendly effort among the learner, peers and teacher. The learner should be aware of the outcomes and goals of the program and the assessment techniques. The assessments, all along the way, are shared with the learner to facilitate growth and development (p. 341).

Gilbert (1992) provides many different types of assessment and evaluation tools including skills checklists, performance critiques, unit tests on a variety of concepts, and an anecdotal form. The directions for using these instruments are clear and simple.

Purcell (1994) noted that "Assessment in dance is a continuous process of evaluating how well the objectives of the learning experience are met." (p. 47) She suggested that the assessment of a dance program had "four views: teacher assessment of the overall effectiveness of the program; teacher assessment of individual student learning; student to student assessment; and self-assessment by the student. The latter three methods can be used to assess students' psychomotor, cognitive, and affective development." (p. 47)

In assessing the overall dance program, Purcell (1994) listed a series of questions that teachers can ask. Some of these questions are as follows:

> Can all the students perform the steps in the dance?
>
> Can all students remember a sequence of steps and perform them without teacher cues? . . .
>
> Can they describe what the steps repesent about the culture in which the dance was designed?
>
> Are they dancing with a sense of joy in the experience? (p. 48)

Questions related to the ability of the students to change directions, move from side to side, maintain spatial formations, relate positively to partners and the whole group were also asked. (p. 48)

Purcell (1994) noted that the second of the four views of assessment included teacher assessment of individual students. This involves individual student learning, in which the teacher monitors a student's individual progress during a single learning experience or over a period of time. The main question posed in this form of assessment is: "What growth do students exhibit in their attitudes of valuing dance, as well as in their abilities to learn, create, and perform dances?" (p. 48)

The third form of assessment was peer assessment which:

> Provides students with an opportunity to respond to the dance and dancers by describing their perceptions, interpretations, and evaluations in a one-to-one relationship or with a small group. Students can develop the criteria for evaluation and the levels of performance, giving them an active role and ownership in their learning (p. 50).

Students evaluate themselves in the fourth form of assessment recommended by Purcell (1994). They assess:

> What they know about dance, how well they learn or create a dance movement, and how they feel about dance. Students evaluate their learning through a variety of activities that include completing a questionnaire, keeping a journal, having a personal conference with the teacher, writing a letter about their experience, or drawing a picture (p. 50).

Wall and Murray (1994) discussed evaluating dance in the following paragraph:

> In dance, we tend to evaluate in terms of the aesthetics of the movement pattern. Since dance is an art form, as well as a physical activity in which equipment is rarely used, we observe how the body moves, and how it is held in stillness. Questions are asked. Was the body shape effective? Was there an appropriate use of tension? Did the children have a clear focus as they traveled? Because dance is a mixture of the physical and the affective, instruments designed to evaluate children's skills need to take into account quantitative (how high? how fast? which body parts?) and the qualitative (how softly? how fluidly?) components. In folk dances and singing games, the stress may be more on the quantitative elements. In creative dance, the qualitative components may be more important. In your dance program, formative techniques are more appropriate than summative ones, and the instrument designed should be criterion referenced (p. 200).

Bennett and Riemer (1995) acknowledged the importance of regular evaluation even though the practice may seem somewhat subjective. They stated that:

> As with all activity and teaching, evaluation is critical to future success in your classes. Rhythmic activities appear more subjective than they actually are. It is possible to remove some of this subjectivity and to collect information.
>
> Rhythmic activities should be evaluated regularly. Students need regular feed-back, as does the teacher (p. 28).

Bennett and Riemer (1995) created two evaluation instruments. The first instrument is a Likert-type scale for teachers to conduct a self-assessment where the teacher answers questions using "Always 5, 4, 3, 2, 1, Never" as choices. The teacher should score an average of 3 or better on all items throughout the year. Among the twelve questions posed are the following samples:

> I use ability grouping to meet individual needs and provide maximum learning opportunities for all in my rhythm and dance classes.
>
> I maximize supplies, equipment, and facilities to keep every student engaged in activity.
>
> I do not repeat the same rhythmic and dance activities without a change in approach or scope (p. 29).

Bennett and Riemer's second instrument is a Rhythmic Assessment Form that can be used by the teacher to assess a student, and/or for student self-evaluation. The three domains (cognitive, affective, and psychomotor) are evaluated in terms of a checklist style using words such as "recognizes," "understands," and "can . . ." perform certain tasks like maintain, mirror, demonstrate, or lead. (p. 30)

"Evaluate means to examine or judge, to assess by critical judgment," according to Joyce (1994, p. 71). She stated that "In dance, the eyes are the tool for evaluation," and expressed the need for the teacher to watch the children closely to see their movements, learn their movement habits, and "judge whether or not they are challening their bodies and moving with variety." (p. 71) At the end of class her "test" is the *good-bye dance* where students are asked to perform certain elements that were included in the lesson that day.

Joyce (1994) encouraged the teacher with the following paragraphs:

> Watch first to see if their bodies are doing the movement you ask for. Then watch to see that their minds are making them do the movement with variety in level, direction, speed, and force. Finally, watch their facial expressions to see if they are dancing with feeling, with spirit, with emotion.
>
> First, accomplish the physical motion with clarity. Your teaching is then adequate. Next, involve their minds with the movement. Your teaching is then challenging. Finally, involve their spirit. Your teaching is then inspirational! (p. 71)

Joyce (1994) realized that:

> Children often like to see their progress in writing. A chart on the wall listing their names vertically and the goals and elements horizontally can help. One teacher I know has such a chart, and the children show her their efforts whenever they are ready. When they do well, she draws a star under the goal or element with five lines. When they do not do well, she draws a part of a star using perhaps three lines. If they even try, she draws at least one line. They can always go back and complete the stars.
>
> An obvious benefit of evaluating the children's progress is that we teachers assess not only our ability to communicate but also our ability to see. The art of seeing is an important adjunct to the art of teaching (pp. 72-73).

Finally, Joyce (1994) expressed the importance of communication in relationship to assessment and evaluation in the following statement:

> We must be able to communicate—to explain verbally what we want from the children—but we must also be able to evaluate—to see and to judge what they have accomplished and how far they have come in relation to the goal (p. 73).

In 1993, the Minnesota Center for Arts Education published the *Dance Education Initiative Curriculum Guide* which was followed by supplemental chapters in 1994 that included "The Art of Dance," "Teaching Dance," and most importantly for this book, "Practical Application of Assessment in Dance." The contents of this supplemental chapter include the following categories:

> Portfolio Assessment in Dance
> A Formula for Assessment
> A Comprehensive Assessment Design
> A "Multi-purpose" Assessment Chart
> Sample Assessment Instruments

Portfolios are fast becoming an important and popular assessment tool. "A portfolio is a collection of student work in various stages of completion, and the assessment records which have been gathered on that work. It represents various types of learning and various aspects of the art discipline." (Mirus, White, & Bucek, 1993, p. 183)

A sampling of materials of *Possible Contents of a Student Portfolio in Dance* listed in the supplemental chapter of the "Practical Application of Assessment in Dance" (Mirus & White, 1994) included items such as [Bold added]:

> **Improvisations, dance studies, and finished dances**—recorded on video, in words, or represented in other media.
> **Journals**—on assigned topics, or open-ended.
> **Dance reviews** by the student[s] about their own dances, or by peers about the dances of fellow students. . . .
> **Rough drafts or notation for dance movement vocabulary**, dance making, dance sharing, or dance inquiry projects.
> **Tests**—matching, essay, true/false, multiple choice, fill in the blank, etc.
> **Rating scales**—especially useful for specific dance skills, evaluated by self, peers, and/or teacher. . . .
> **Written reports**—on books students have read, interviews they have conducted, events or processes they have experienced (p. 1).

In this supplemental chapter an excellent formula for assessment was presented. This formula provides guidance to teachers in terms of the components of assessment:

Assessment =
Outcome Statements
+
Learning Experiences
+
Assessment Method
(Instrument + Who Does What)
+
Criteria
+
Evidence

Mirus, White, and Bucek (1993) discussed important aspects of outcome-based education and how it fits into assessment and evaluation. They stated that:

> Outcome-based education focuses on the student's response to educational experiences rather than on a menu of topics that the student will encounter within specified time-blocks. In Outcome-based education, both curriculum planning and assessment are guided by statements that characterize expected achievement by students (p. 137).

In the *Dance Education Initiative Currciulum Guide,* Mirus, White, and Bucek (1993) said "statements of desirable and expected student achievement are expressed as Goals of Dance Learning, Learner Outcome Statements, and Sample Instructional Objectives." They identified each one of these areas as follows:

> **Goals of Dance Learning** are encompassing statements that characterize the abilities, knowledge, and attitudes attained through continuing and thorough dance study. Progress toward each Goal results from broadbased achievement in learning across the Dance Discipline.
>
> *(continued)*

Learner Outcome Statements are more specific than Goals. Achievement of many Learner Outcomes in each of the Discipline Areas (Dance Movement Vocabulary, Dance Making, Dance Sharing, and Dance Inquiry) will contribute to increasingly sophisticated achievement of the Goals.

Instructional Objectives are still more specific. They are statements of observable student response to the learning experiences presented in instructional units and lessons. Teachers will find that they can create many Instructional Objectives that will lead toward the achievement of each Learner Outcome. Instructional Objectives may thus be thought of as "sub-outcomes."

Student achieve **Goals**
    through the mastery of **Learner Outcomes.**
      Students achieve **Learner Outcomes**
        through the mastery of **Instructional Objectives.**(p. 137)

"The Learner Outcomes and sample Instructional Objectives in this Guide are stated in terms of what the student will *Know, Do, Value,* and *Create,* as a result of education in dance." (p. 138). These learner outcomes and instructional objectives are then linked to four major areas of learning that include Dance Movement Vocabulary, Dance Making, Dance Sharing, and Dance Inquiry. Therefore, "through instruction and practice in dance in these four areas, students KNOW, DO, VALUE, and CREATE certain aspects in each area." These four areas are defined as follows [Bold added]:

Dance Movement Vocabulary is human movement explored or practiced as dance.

Dance Making is creating dance shapes, movements, phrases, studies, and complete dances.

Dance Sharing is communicating with others through dancing, responding to, and recording dance.

Dance Inquiry is asking questions, researching and theorizing about dance as it is experienced and expressed in a variety of cultural, social, and historical contexts. (pp. 145-149)

As a sample, the first (of several) statements in each category (know, do, value, and create) was selected from the Learner Outcome Statements for the area of Dance Movement Vocabulary:

> **Through instruction and practice in dance, students**
>
> **KNOW :**
> - ¥ that dance movement vocabulary can be developed from any human movement.
>
> **DO :**
> - ¥ explore and extend their personal range of movement capabilties.
>
> **VALUE :**
> - ¥ dance movement and health practices that respect the body as an instrument of expression.
>
> **CREATE :**
> - ¥ create personal movement vocabulary in response to a variety of images, ideas, feelings, themes, and structures (p. 145).

Seven innovative assessment instruments with charts and easy-to-follow directions for using them are included in the supplemental chapter on "Practical Application of Assessment in Dance" (1994). Authors, Mirus and White, suggested that such assessments can become part of a student's portfolio. Teachers would be wise to order these materials from the Minnesota Center for Arts Education. (The address is located in the resources at the end of the book.)

Another important contribution to the area of assessment in dance was provided by *The National Standards for Arts Education —Dance, Music, Theatre, and Visual Arts* (1994). This publication is another milestone in moving the arts toward credibility. In the *Summary Statement,* the Standards are presented as follows:

> These *National Standards for Arts Education* are a statement of what every young American should know and be able to do in four arts disciplines—dance, music, theatre, and the visual arts. Their scope is grades K-12, and they speak to both content and achievement. The standards are one outcome of the education reform effort generated in the 1980's, which emerged in several states and attained nationwide visibility with the publication of *A Nation at Risk* in 1983. . . . Six national education goals were announced in 1990. . . . With the passage of the *Goals 2000: Educate America Act,* the national goals are written into law, naming the arts as a core, academic subject—as important to education as English, mathematics, history, civics and government, geography, science, and foreign language. (Monograph, pp. 1-2)

"What Students Should Know and Be Able to Do in the Arts," is the basis for the development of the National Standards for Arts Education (1994).

> Essentially, the Standards ask that student should know and be able to do the following by the time they have completed secondary school:
>
> *They should be able to communicate at a basic level in the four arts disciplines*—dance, music, theatre, and the visual arts. This includes knowledge and skills in the use of the basic vocabularies, materials, tools, techniques, and intellectual methods of each arts discipline.
>
> *They should be able to communicate proficiently in at least one art form*, including the ability to define and solve artistic problems with insight, reason, and technical proficiency.
>
> * *They should be able to develop and present basic analyses of works of art* from structural, historical, and cultural perspectives, and from combinations of those perspectives. This includes the ability to understand and evaluate work in the various arts disciplines.
>
> * *They should have an informed acquaintance with exemplary works of art from a variety of cultures and historical periods*, and a basic understanding of historical development in the arts disciplines, across the arts as a whole, and within cultures.
>
> * *They should be able to relate various types of arts knowledge and skills within and across the arts disciplines.* This includes mixing and matching competencies and understandings in art-making, history and culture, and analysis in any arts-related project.
>
> As a result of developing these capabilities, students can arrive at their own knowledge, beliefs, and values for making personal and artistic decisions. In other terms, they can arrive at a broad-based, well-grounded understanding of the nature, value, and meaning of the arts as a part of their own humanity. (pp. 18-19)

The format of the National Standards is the presentation of standards for each of the arts disciplines (Dance, Music, Theatre, Visual Arts) in blocks of Grades K-4, Grades 5-8, and Grades 9-12. The format of using the following two types of standards is consistent throughout [Bold added]:

> *Content Standards* specify what students should know and be able to do in the arts disciplines
>
> *Achievement Standards* specify the understandings and levels of achievement that students are expected to attain in the competencies, for each of the arts, at the completion of grades 4, 8, and 12. (p. 18)

Specific competencies are listed within each of the disciplines that "the arts education community, nationwide, believes are essential for every student. Although the statement of any specific competency in any of the arts disciplines necessarily focuses on one part of that discipline, the Standards stress that all the competencies are interdependent." (National Standards for Arts Education, p. 18)

One example of how the Standards were set up was selected from the first set of standards in Dance, Grades K-4. [An asterisk * indicates that the terms were defined in the dance glossary at the end of the Standards.]

> **Content Standard:** Identifying and demonstrating movement elements and skills in performing dance
>
> **Achievement Standard:**
> Students
>
> a. accurately demonstrate nonlocomotor/*axial movements (such as bend, twist, stretch, swing)
>
> b. accurately demonstrate eight basic *locomotor movements (such as walk, run, hop, jump, leap, gallop, slide, and skip), traveling forward, backward, sideward, diagonally, and turning
>
> c. create shapes at low, middle, and high *levels
>
> d. demonstrate the ability to define and maintain *personal space
>
> e. demonstrate movements in straight and curved pathways
>
> f. demonstrate accuracy in moving to a musical beat and responding to changes in tempo
>
> g. demonstrate *kinesthetic awareness, concentration, and focus in performing movement skills
>
> h. attentively observe and accurately describe the *action (such as skip, gallop) and movement elements (such as *levels, directions) in a brief movement study (p. 23)

The same seven content standards are listed for each of the three grade blocks. Of course, many more achievement standards are listed at the higher grades. Appendix 2 of the Standards provides Outlines of Sequential Learning that illustrate Content Standard One followed by the achievement standards for each grade block. This chart makes possible the scanning of achievement standards from K-12. The high school levels of achievement are listed as **Grades 9-12 Proficient** (indicating that the student has achieved the basic level of understanding and skill) and **Grades 9-12 Advanced** (indicating that the student has progressed beyond the basic understandings and skill achievement).

In their article, "What National Dance Standards Mean to You," Howe and Kimball (1994) discussed the history of the development of educational reform that ultimately resulted in these standards. They also discussed the fact that:

> The United States is one of the few industrialized nations without a national curriculum. The standards present a solution to this issue; they give national shape to—and yet retain state and local control over[—]decision making with regard to curricular specifics (p. 38).

Howe & Kimball (1994) pointed out that adopting and implementing these standards are voluntary and that each state will choose whether or not to adopt these standards, followed up by providing the necessary resources to create a program to meet each standard.

The task remains, now, for us to implement the National Standards for Arts Education in our classes at the local level. We must encourage our colleagues and school and community administrators to adopt and help implement these Standards as we move toward the year 2000 and beyond, as we strive to develop excellence in dance, as well as the other art forms in our lives and in the lives of our students.

CONCLUSION

In pondering "the good old days"—when we simply danced without thoughts of outcomes, assessment, and evaluations racing through our minds (mostly because we simply did not know about these "things")—one wonders how far dance could have come and would have come by now, IF we would have had the foresight, insight, and where-with-all to discern what we wanted (our goals) and then assess and evaluate our achievements. Would dance be more highly respected and valued now? Would dance have taken its rightful place in the curriculum and become a partner with other disciplines like mathematics, science, and history? Would we have become more proficient students of dance and more proficient teachers of dance?

These questions are difficult to answer without 20/20 hindsight. But if we "jump on the assessment/evaluation bandwagon now," for the right reasons, we will become involved in the process of answering these questions for the future. Maybe in a few years, we will not be wondering—we will know what we want to achieve, what has been achieved, and what we can predict for future achievements in dance and all of its facets—education, appreciation, art, performance, recreation, exercise, and therapy.

SUMMARY

This chapter discussed the important topic of assessment and evaluation in dance. Viewpoints of various authors concerning this subject were presented. The importance, necessity, and relevance of assessment and evaluation were discussed, followed by a brief description of various assessment and evaluation tools.

A few details about The National Standards for Arts Education were presented along with a discussion of the importance of these standards to dance. A challenge was issued to teachers and administrators to adopt and implement these standards in order to produce students who are well grounded in dance and the other arts. Everyone, no matter what age, ability, or culture has a right to dance.

References

Ayob, Salmah. (1986). *An Examination of Purpose Concept in Creative Dance for Children.* Unpublished doctoral dissertation, University of Wisconsin, Madison.

Beech, Tamara. (October, 1995). Common Toys Make Uncommon Classes. *Dance Teacher Now, 17*(8), 77-79.

Bennett, John Price, & Riemer, Pamela Coughenour. (1995). *Rhythmic Activities and Dance.* Champaign, IL: Human Kinetics.

Boorman, Joyce. (1969). *Creative Dance in The First Three Grades.* New York, NY: David McKay.

Brooks, Nancy Jean. (1978). *A Creative Movement Workbook for Classroom Teachers.* Missoula, MT: Center for Continuing Education, University of Montana.

Dance Grades K-12. A Guide for Idaho Public Schools. (1991). Boise, ID: Idaho State Department of Education.

Dance as Education. (1977). Reston, VA: National Dance Association/ American Alliance for Health, Physical Education, Recreation and Dance.

Dorien, Margery. (1978). *Ethnic Stories for Children to Dance.* San Mateo, CA: BBB Associates.

Dunkin, Anne. (April, 1988). Movement Experiences for Young Students. *Dance Teacher Now, 10* (3), 30-32.

Fleming, Gladys Andrews. (1976). *Creative Rhythmic Movement. Boys and Girls Dancing.* Englewood Cliffs, NJ: Prentice Hall

Gardner, Howard. (1983). *Frames of Mind. The Theory of Multiple Intelligences.* New York, NY: Basic Books.

Gilbert, Anne Green. (1992). *Creative Dance for All Ages: A Conceptual Approach.* Reston, VA: National Dance Association/American Alliance for Health, Physical Education, Recreation and Dance.

Graham, George, Holt/Hale, Shirley Ann, & Parker, Melissa. (1993). *Children Moving. A Reflective Approach to Teaching Physical Education* (3rd ed.). Mountain View, CA: Mayfield Publishing Co.

Hall, J. Tillman, Sweeny, Nancy Hall, & Esser, Jody Hall. (1980). *Physical Education in the Elementary School.* Santa Monica, CA: Goodyear.

Harris, Jane A., Pittman, Anne, M., & Waller, Marlys S. (1994). *Dance A While* (7th ed.). New York, NY: Macmillan.

Howe, Dianne S., & Kimball, Mary Maitland. (September, 1994). What National Dance Standards Mean to You. *Dance Teacher Now, 16* (7), 32-41, 44-45.

Humphrey, James H. (1987). *Child Development and Learning Through Dance.* New York, NY: AMS Press.

Joyce, Mary. (1994). *First Steps in Teaching Creative Dance to Children* (3rd ed.). Mountain View, CA: Mayfield Publishing Co.

Joyce, Mary. (1980). *First Steps in Teaching Creative Dance to Children* (2nd ed.). Palo Alto, CA: Mayfield Publishing Co.

Laban, Rudolf. (1975). *Modern Educational Dance* (3rd ed.). London, England: Macdonald & Evans Ltd. (Revised by Lisa Ullmann).

Lockhart, Aileen, & Pease, Esther E. (1973). *Modern Dance. Building and Teaching Lessons* (4th ed.). Dubuque, IA: Wm. C. Brown.

Mettler, Barbara. (1960). *Materials of Dance as a Creative Art Activity.* Tucson, AZ: Mettler Studios.

Mirus, Judith, & White, Elena. (1994). *Practical Application of Assessment in Dance. A Supplemental Chapter to the Dance Education Initiative Curriculum Guide.* Golden Valley, MN: Minnesota Center for Arts Education.

Mirus, Judith, White, Elena, & Bucek, Loren E. (1993). *Dance Education Initiative Curriculum Guide.* Golden Valley, MN: Minnesota Center for Arts Education.

Murray, Ruth Lovell. (1975). *Dance in Elementary Education* (3rd ed.). New York, NY: Harper & Row.

Nash, Grace C. (1972). *Verses and Movement. Music With Children* (6th Printing). Scottsdale, Arizona: Swartout Enterprises. (now The Grace Nash Publications)

National Standards for Arts Education. (1994). Reston, VA: Music Educators National Conference

National Standards for Arts Education. Summary Statement. (1994). Reston, VA: Music Educators National Conference.

Pre-school Curriculum Guidelines for Malaysia. A seminar paper. (1972). Kuala Lumpur, Malaysia: Ministry of Education.

Purcell, Theresa M. (November 9, 1995). *Creating New Folk Dances for Today's Generation.* Paper presented at the meeting of the New Jersey Association for Health, Physical Education, Recreation and Dance.

Purcell, Theresa M. (1994). *Teaching Children Dance. Becoming a Master Teacher.* Champaign, IL: Human Kinetics.

Purcell, Theresa M. (1990). *Creating Contemporary Folk Dances.* Unpublished paper.

Raftis, Alkis (Ed.). (1991). *Dance in Poetry. An International Anthology of Poems on Dance.* Princeton, NJ: Princeton Book Company.

Riggs, Maida L. (Ed.). (1980). *Movement Education for Pre-school Children.* Reston, VA: American Alliance for Health, Physical Education, Recreation and Dance.

Russell, Joan. (1968). *Creative Dance in the Primary School.* New York, NY: Praeger.

Seefeldt, Vern. (1980). *Guidelines for Pre-school Children.* NASPE Presidents' Council on Physical Education and Sports, February 1-2, 1980. Reston, VA: American Alliance for Health, Physical Education, Recreation and Dance.

Stinson, Susan W. (1991). Promising Practices in Arts Education Assessment. In L. Overby (Ed.), *Early Childhood Creative Arts.* Proceedings of the International Early Childhood Creative Arts Conference. Los Angeles, CA, December 6-9, 1990. Reston, VA: National Dance Association/American Alliance for Health, Physical Education, Recreation and Dance.

Stinson, Sue. (1988). *Dance for Young Children. Finding the Magic in Movement.* Reston, VA: American Alliance for Health, Physical Education, Recreation and Dance.

Sullivan, Molly. (1982). *Feeling Strong, Feeling Free: Movement Exploration for or Young Children.* Washington, D.C.: National Association for the Education of Young Children.

Tobias, Anne. (1994, January). SounDance. Fostering the Children of the Second City. *Dance Magazine, LXVIII* (1), 76-79.

Wall, Jennifer, & Murray, Nancy. (1994). *Children & Movement. Physical Education in the Elementary School* (2nd ed.). Madison, WI/ Dubuque, IA: Brown & Benchmark.

Warren, Jean. (1984). *Movement Time.* Palo Alto, CA: Monday Morning Books.

Waterman, Elizabeth. (1936). *The Rhythm Book. A Manual for Teachers of Children.* New York, NY: A. S. Barnes.

Weikart, Phyllis S. (1982). *Teaching Movement & Dance.* Ypsilanti, MI: The High/Scope Press.

Zirulnik, Ann. (1979). Body Parts. In J. Abels & S. McColl (Eds.), *Creative Dance Starters.* East Lansing, MI: Michigan Dance Association.

RESOURCES

Selected organizations, dance book publishers, music sources, dance videos, books, articles and monographs, periodicals, and internet information have been provided to assist teachers in locating further information about dance.

SELECTED ORGANIZATIONS THAT PROMOTE DANCE

The National Dance Association
American Alliance for Health, Physical Education, Recreation and Dance
1900 Association Drive
Reston, Virginia 20191-1599
Telephone: 703-476-3436   FAX: 703-476-9527
Publications: 1-800-321-0789
E-mail: nda@aahperd.org

Dance and the Child International (daCi)
USA Representative as of 1996
Sara Lee Gibb
293 Richards Building
Brigham Young University
Provo, Utah 84602

Canadian Representative as of 1996
Ann Kipling-Brown
Faculty of Education
University of Regina
Regina
Saskatchewan S4S OA2 Canada

National Association for the Education of Young Children (NAEYC)
1509 16th Street NW
Washington, D.C. 20036-1426
Telephone: 1-800-424-2460

California Dance Educator's Association
Midge Kretchner (work: Lick-Wilmerding High
School 415-333-4021)
1996-1997 President of CDEA
Home: 415-885-6416
Fax: 415-885-0121

Dance Educators Association of Washington (DEAW)
12577 Densmore Avenue North
Seattle, Washington 98133
(Monthly newsletters that include valuable and useful information including lesson plans for all ages, as well as association news. Write for membership information.)

Maryland Council for Dance
Washington College
300 Washington Avenue
Chestertown, MD 21620-1197

Also check your own locale for state and regional dance organizations, or contact the National Dance Association for information about organizations or arts councils in your area.

DANCE BOOK PUBLISHERS

eddie bowers publishing, inc.
2600 Jackson Street
Dubuque, IA 52001
Telephone: 1-319-588-2411

Mayfield Publishing Company
1240 Villa Street
Mountain View, CA 94041
Telephone: 1-415-960-3222

Minnesota Center for Arts Education
6125 Olson Memorial Highway,
Golden Valley, MN 55422
Phone: 1-800-657-3515 or (612) 591-4700
Contact the center for videos and publications that are for sale including the new *Dance Education Initiative Curriculum Guide.* 2nd Ed. (1996)

Princeton Book Company Publishers
12 West Delaware Avenue
Pennington, New Jersey 08534
Telephone: 1-800-220-7149

The Dance Mart
P. O. Box 994
Teaneck, NJ 07666
This company handles rare books, magazines, autograph material, and other collectibles in dance. Most items are out of print.

Zephyr Press
P.O. Box 66006
Tucson, Arizona 85728-6006
Telephone: 502-322-5090 Ext. 102
Fax: 520-323-9402

MUSIC SOURCES

Educational Activities
P.O. Box 87
Baldwin, New York 11510
1-800-645-3739

Kimbo Educational
Dept. X
P.O. Box 477
Long Branch, New Jersey 07740-0477
1-800-631-2187

Eric Chappelle
Ravenna Ventures, Inc.
4756 University Village Pl. NE, #117
Seattle, Washington 98105
Telephone (206) 522-7799

(As of 1995, Chappelle has composed two albums——Contrast & Continuum Volumes I and II. Especially created for creative dance, the majority of pieces on these volumes feature contrasts in tempo, texture and other music elements which correspond to dance elements. Each CD contains a booklet with ideas for movements and dance themes.)

DANCE VIDEOS

Ballroom Dance, American Style. (1 hr. 45 min. video by Shirley Rushing and Patrick McMillan) contains the basic steps and 70 variations for 10 dances. ($39.95) Contact eddie bowers publishing, inc., 2600 Jackson Street, Dubuque, IA 52001 (1-319-588-2411)

For information about the following videos (plus many more dance videos) contact Princeton Book Company, Publishers, Pennington, NJ, 1-800-220-7149.

Creative Movement. A Step Towards Intelligence for Children Ages 2-8 (80 min., color, 1993)

Dance and Grow. Developmental Activities for Three through Eight Year Olds. Written and directed by Betty Rowen. (50 min., color, 1994)

DANCING. (1993). A complete "dance package" that includes: <u>8 videotapes</u> VHS (58 min. each) (about $200) <u>A companion book: Dancing</u> by Gerald Jonas published by Harry N. Abrams, NY.

The *Teacher's Resource Guide* was designed to accompany the video series. Designed to supplement secondary school social studies, world cultures, and dance curricula, the materials include program summaries, before- and after-viewing activites, student activity sheets, research and performance projects, a bibliography and a poster for classroom use. To obtain a copy, please write to: DANCING Resource Guide, P.O. Box 245, Little Falls, NJ 07424-9876.

The videos, numbered 1-8, are boxed individually and come in a large box to store the set. The descriptions presented are abbreviated from materials sent prior to the viewing of the series which aired on PBS nationwide in 1993.

1. **The Power of Dance.** Jacques d'Amboise teaches children dance. Russian dancers, Indian gurus, American song-and-dance men, and others talk about the quest for that one perfect moment when actions speak louder than words.

2. **Lord of the Dance.** In the Hindu myth of creation the cosmos came into being by divine dance. What cultural beliefs have shaped the great traditions of sacred and secular dance? A look at Christian attitudes about dance, and a visit to Nigeria to view a religious group dancing.

3. **Sex and Social Dance.** Polynesians were shocked to see respectable Europeans locked in an embrace while dancing. We all dance, but what social values and ideals infuse the dances that we do?

4. **Dance at Court.** In the contemporary courts of Japan, Java, Ghana, dance thrives as a symbol of order, a model of correct behavior, and a source of reliable information about who's who in the corridors of power.

5. **New Worlds, New Forms.** From the Samba in Rio to the Lindy-hop in Harlem, cultural collisions have shaped the popular dances in the Americas, where dance has become a medium for cultural fusion among Africans and Europeans.

6. **Dance Centerstage.** From the Imperial capital of St. Petersburg, where classical ballet was developed, to the streets of Kyoto, where Kabuki emerged, this tape traces the meanings behind these classical forms.

7. **The Individual and Tradition.** This program examines the art of "making it new" in the work of Isadora Duncan, Martha Graham, Katherine Dunham, George Balanchine, Twyla Tharp, Eiko and Koma, Sardono Kusumo, Garth Fagan.

8. **Dancing In One World.** At the Los Angeles Festival, an international gathering of young dancers captures the tensions and aspirations of our "global village" on the brink of a new century.

The following Dancing Colors videotapes were created and produced by Emily Day and can be purchased by contacting: Dancing Colors, P.O. Box 61, Langley, WA 98620. Phone: 360-221-5989.

Dancing Colors: Scarves for Dance Therapy, Education, Performance and Ritual, 35 min. VHS $29.95

Dancing Colors Take to the Air (1992) 55 min. VHS $39.95 Introductory special: Both for $59.95. Write or telephone for a free catalog.

Gill, Sue, & Hohendorf, Diane V. (1991). **Fundamental Dance Signs.** Reston, VA: National Dance Association/American Alliance for Health, Physical Education, Recreation and Dance. (21 min. $25) Signs in communicating with the hearing impaired.

Old Friends. An Intergenerational Approach to Dance. (25 min. video) about dance workshops presented by college students, and Josie Metal-Corbin to older adults. Contact Josie Metal-Corbin, the University of Nebraska, Omaha 68182.

A Very Special Dance (15 min. movie) highlights special populations and the dances they created with the guidance of Anne Riordan. Rent from the National Dance Association.

DANCE ON THE INTERNET

Afterimages is a quarterly newsletter of performing arts documentation and preservation edited by Leslie Hansen Kopp and published by :

Preserve, Inc.
P.O. Box 743
Falls Church, VA 22040-0743
Telephone: 703-573-9580   FAX: 703-573-9581
e-mail: **Preserve_Inc@msn.com**.

Dance on the Internet was featured in the Spring and Summer 1995 publication of *Afterimages*. A description of connecting to the Internet, tools available, subscribing to Listserv (which allows access to discussion groups in a wide variety of dance forms) getting into the Dance Collection at the New York Public Library, and World Wide Web resources was provided. The information furnished below was taken from *Aterimages, 2* (2 and 3), Spring and Summer 1995 (pp. 7-8).

Here are Dance Listserv Addresses:

National Dance Association has a listserv address. Here is how to get on to that list: open your e-mail and in the space for
        To: **listserv@msu.edu.**
Go to the body of the e-mail document and enter:
        subscribe ndalist your name.
You should then be on the NDA list. If there is a problem of getting on this list contact the NDA office via e-mail, telephone or fax which is listed in the Resources under Organizations.

amia-l@ukcc.uky.edu (Association of Moving Image Archivists)
ballet-modern-dance@netcom.com (Ballet and modern dance)
ballroom@athena.mit.edu (Ballroom dancing)
dance-hc@cunyvm.cuny.edu (The Dance Heritage Coalition's Clearinghouse)
dance-tech@ohio-state.edu (Dance and technology)
dldg-l@iubvm.usc.indiana.edu (The Dance Librarians Discussion Group)
rendance-l@morgan.uc.mun.ca (Renaissance dance)
morris-l@suvm.acs.syr.edu (Morris dance)
strathspey-l@maath.uni-frankfurt.de (Scottish country dancing)
tango-l@mitvma.mit.edu (Argentine tango)
uk-dance@tqmcomms.co.uk (Dance-music-culture in the United Kingdom)

DANCE ON THE INTERNET: TELNET TO THE NYPL DANCE COLLECTION CATALOG

Clearly the foremost collection of dance materials in the world, The Dance Collection of The New York Public Library is a treasure house of information on virtually every type and aspect of dance. The collection includes some 40,000 book volumes, seventy-five periodical subscriptions, 355,000 manuscripts, 1,000 microfilm reels, 9,000 videotapes and films, 1,600 oral history tapes, 200,00 clippings, 2,050 original stage and costume designs, 250,000 photographs, 150,400 negatives, 6,000 prints, 4,450 posters, 92,000 programs , and 2,210 scrapbooks.

The NYPL Dance Collection on-line catalog is available over the Internet as well as in the reading room and the Performing Arts Library at Lincoln Center. To access the Dance Collection Catalog, use the following address:

telnet nyplgate.nypl.org (or 192.94.250.2)
login: nypl
password: nypl

Once successfully logged on, you will see the menu screen. Select the Dance Collection Catalog or the Research Libraries Catalog.

The online (telnet) access to the NYPL Dance Collection Catalog may, at some point in the future, change to a different system. When this event will take place, no one knows, however, readers should be familiar with the current point of access to such a valuable collection. After you have experienced NYPLnet, you can telnet to the:

Library of Congress   **locis.loc.gov**
Harvard Theatre Collection   **hollis.harvard.edu**

Other valuable information from *Afterimages* that could be of assistance follows.

SELECTED INTERNET ADDRESSES

Canada Council — funding grant programs for the dance field.
    http://WWW.ffa.ucalgary.ca/cc/dance.html
WWW Virtual Dance Library
    http://www.tmn.com/Artswire/www/dance/dance.html
National Ballet of Canada
    http://www.ffa.ucalgary.ca/nbc/nbc_main.html
Boston Ballet
    http://www.arts-online.com/bbalet.html
San Francisco Ballet
    http://www-leland.stanford.edu/~rbeal/sfb.html
Jacques D'Amboise (brief audio clip from a lecture about time/space given by D'Amboise and recorded live at the Celebrity Lecture in the Midwest)

http://web.msu.edu/lecture/amboise.html
The Kennedy Center's premier Web site for arts education is **Arts Edge**
http://artsedge.kennedy-center.org/
The Kennedy Center Education Program
http://gopher.tmn.com:70/11/NAEIN/menu.b17

These are just a few addresses to begin exploring dance over the Internet. For more information about Dance and the Internet, contact Preserve and request a copy of *Afterimages* Spring/Summer 1995 for more details and get on their mailing list.

"Getting Caught in the 'Web'," by Luke Kahlich (July 1966) described various World Wide Web (www) sites and how to begin accessing this information on the computer. He listed a wide variety of dance topics with addresses and brief descriptions of information to be accessed at each site. See: Impulse. The International Journal of Dance Science, Medicine, and Education, 4(3), 181-86.

ARTS EDUCATION

ArtsEdNet is a new electronic information resource for the arts education community established by the Getty Center in Santa Monica, California. The purpose of ArtsEdNet is to talk, learn, inspire, and draw on rich library online resources when needed. Here are three ways to get in touch with the Getty Center:

Mail:
The Getty Education Institute for the Arts
1200 Getty Center Drive, Suite 600
Los Angeles, CA 90049-1683
Phone: 310-440-7315
FAX: 310-440-7704
Internet: **http://www.artsednet.getty.edu**

SELECTED BOOKS

(in addition to those in the References)

Beal, Rayma, & Berryman-Miller, Sherrill (Eds.). (1988). *Dance for the Older Adult. Focus on Dance XI.* Reston, VA: National Dance Association/American Alliance for Health, Physical Education, Recreation and Dance.

Canner, Norma, & Klebanoff, Harriet. (1975) *. . . and a time to dance.* Boston, MA; Plays, Inc. ("A sensitive exposition of the use of creative movement with children with disabilities.")

Corbin, David, & Metal-Corbin, Josie (1983). *Reach for It! A Handbook of Exercise and Dance Activities for Older Adults*. Dubuque, IA: eddie bowers publishing inc.

Dance Education in the Vancouver Schools: K-12 Curriculum. (1990). Vancouver, WA: Office of Visual and Performing Arts, Vancouver School District.

Dance Education Initiative Curriculum Guide (2nd ed.). (1996). Minneapolis, MN: Minnesota Center for Arts Education.

Dance Curricula Guidelines K-12. (1991). Reston, VA: National Dance Association.

Gilbert, Anne Green. (1977). *Teaching the Three Rs Through Movement Experiences*. New York, NY: Macmillan

Herman, Gail, & Hollingsworth, Patricia. (1992). *Kinetic Kaleidoscope. Exploring Movement and Energy in the Visual Arts*. Tucson, AZ: Zephyr Press.

Heth, Charlotte (Ed.). (1992). *Native American Dance: Ceremonies and Social Traditions*. Washington, D.C.: Smithsonian.

Landalf, Helen, and Gerke, Pamela. (1996). *Movement Stories for Children Ages 3-6*. Lyme, NH: Smith and Kraus, Inc.

Levine, Mindy. (1994). *Widening the Circle. Toward a New Vision for Dance Education*. Washington, D.C.: Dance/USA.

McGreevy-Nichols, Susan, and Scheff, Helene. (1995). *Building Dances. A Guide to Putting Movements Together*. Pennington, NJ: Princeton Book Co. Publishers.

Nahumck, Nadia Chikovsky. (1980). *Dance Curriculum Resource Guide. Comprehensive Dance Education for Secondary Schools*. New York: NY: American Dance Guild.

Pica, Rae. (1991). *Special Themes for Moving & Learning*. Champaign, IL: Human Kinetics.

Rushing, Shirley and McMillan, Patrick. (1997). *Ballroom Dance: American Style*. Dubuque, IA: eddie bowers publishing, inc.

Weiler, Virginia, Mass, Joan Mills, and Nirschl, Evelyn. (1988). *A Guide to Curriculum Planning in Dance*. Madison, WI: Wisconsin Department of Public Instruction.

SELECTED CHILDREN'S BOOKS

Aardema, Verna. (1976). *A Masai Tale. Who's in Rabbit's House?* New York, NY: The Dial Press.

Getz, Arthur. (1980.) *Humphrey, The Dancing Pig.* New York, NY: Dial Press.

Hautzig, Deborah. (1983). *The Story of the Nutcracker Ballet.* New York, NY: Random House.

McKissick, Patricia. (1988). *Mirandy and Brother Wind.* New York, NY: Knopf.

My Ballet Book. A Write-in-Me Book for Young Dancers. (1993). Glenview, IL: Harper Collins.

Thaler, Mike. (1989). *The Teacher from the Black Lagoon .* New York, NY: Scholastic Inc.

Many books are available for use with children and creative movement and dance activities. Authors such as Maurice Sendak, Rachel Isadora, and others have written books that are easily located in any library.

SELECTED ARTICLES AND MONOGRAPHS

ARTICLES

Beal, Rayma K. (1993, March/April). Issues in Dance Education. *Arts Education Policy Review 94* (4), 35-39.

Clements, Rhonda L. , and Oosten, Maureen. (1995, March). Creating and Implementing Preschool Movement Narratives. *Journal of Physical Education, Recreation and Dance, 66* (3), 24-29.

Downey, Vicki. (1995, November/December). Expressing Ideas Through Gesture, Time, and Space. *Journal of Physical Education,Recreation and Dance, 66* (9), 24-29.

Kahlich, Luke. (1996). Getting Caught in the Web. *Impulse. The International Journal of Dance Science, Medicine, and Education, 4*(3), 181-86.

Pica, Rae. (1995). What to Expect from 5 to 8 Year Olds. *Dance Teacher Now, 17* (3), 54-61.

Dance Dynamics Features in the *Journal of Physical Education, Recreation and Dance,* referred to hereafter as *JOPERD*.

Shuker, Virginia, and Brightman, Peg (Eds.). (1992). Dance Education K-12—Theory into Practice (Part I). *JOPERD, 63* (9), 37-57.
(Article titles include: Introduction, Constructing a Child Centered Dance Curriculum; A Conceptual approach to Studio Dance, Pre K-12; Creating Dances and Dance Instruction—An Integrated-Arts Approach; and Toward a Vision of Dance Education for Children.)

Shuker, Virginia, and Brightman, Peg (Eds.) . (1993). Dance education K-12—Theory into practice (Part II). *JOPERD, 64* (5), 41-59, 70-71.
(Articles include: Introduction; Learning Through the Arts; Co-operative Learning and Dance Education, and Voices From Schools—The Significance of Relationships to Public School Dance Students.)

Kerr-Berry, Julie A. (Feature Ed.) (1994). African Dance. Enhancing the Curriculum. *Journal of Physical Education, Recreation and Dance, 65* (5), 25-47.
(Contains six articles focusing on African dance in the schools, including an article titled, "Teaching Creative Dance—An Afrocentric Perspective" by Connie Vandarakis-Fenning.)

MONOGRAPHS

Dance Education—What Is It? Why Is It Important? (1991). Reston, VA: The National Dance Association/American Alliance for Health, Physical Education, Recreation and Dance.

SELECTED PERIODICALS

Dance Magazine
Dance Teacher Now
Dance & the Arts
Dance Research Journal
Dance Chronicle
Impulse
Viltis

DUPLICATE LESSONS FROM CHAPTERS 4 THROUGH 7

<table>
<tr><td></td><td>Time Allotment_____</td></tr>
</table>

Outline of Lesson Plan One
"My Body Moves"

Grade/Age_____

Number of Students_____

Unit title: *The Body* Lesson title: *My Body Moves* Date:	Props/Materials: Visual Aids: *Pictures (Poster) of people moving*
Objectives 1. *identify body parts* 2. *explore ways of moving body parts* 3. *explore shapes + levels* 4. *create a movement pattern (shape-movement-shape)*	Equipment: *Drum, Cassette / CD Player* Accompaniment: *music, voice percussion*

Activities of the Lesson	Formation	Time
WARM UPS 1. *Heads, shoulders, knees, toes* 2. *Stretch, bend, "hang over," curl up* 3. *Twist - snap - stamp - clap* 4. *Walk - forward, backward, freeze*	*Circle: sitting standing scattered*	*5 min.*
MOVEMENT EXPLORATION ACTIVITIES *Show pictures - identify body parts, movements, shapes + levels* *"How many ways can body parts move when: lying down, sitting, kneeling, standing* *Poem "Never Bump"* *Walk, fwd, backward - freeze in shape at high, medium, low levels*	*Sitting in a group, facing teacher.* *Circle* *Scattered*	*5 - 7 min.*

GATHERING ACTIVITY (*Shape-Movement-Shape*)
 Combination:
   SHAPE: *low-stretched*   *4 counts*
   MOVEMENT: *walk forward*   *8 counts*
   SHAPE: *high-twisted*   *4 counts*
 Add
   MOVEMENT: *walk backwards*   *8 counts*
   SHAPE: *your own*   *8 counts*
 Show + Share
	Scattered	*10 - 15 min.*

RELAXATION (1) *Breathe, curl down + up*. (2) *Neck circles* (3) *Tight + loose* (4) *Stretch + relax* (5) *Slow music for 30-60 seconds*	*Circle: Sitting* *Lying on back*	*5 min.*
Evaluation of the lesson: 1. What went well? 2. What can be improved?		

Time Allotment_____

Grade/Age_____

Outline of Lesson Plan Two
"Copycat"

Number of Students_____

Unit title: *The Body* Lesson title: *Copycat* Date:	**Props/Materials:** **Visual Aids:** Diagram on chalkboard *Swing*
Objectives 1. *explore body parts swinging* 2. *explore body shapes* 3. *copy shapes* 4. *create a movement combination*	**Equipment:** *Drum,* *cassette/CD player* **Accompaniment:** *Voice, music*

Activities of the Lesson	**Formation**	**Time**
WARM UPS 1. *arm swings* 2. *leg swings* 3. *slides - right + left*	*Standing* *Scattered*	*5 min.*
MOVEMENT EXPLORATION ACTIVITIES *Follow-the-leader - copy shapes* *Explore levels + shapes* *Repeat activity*	*Circle:* *Standing*	*5 - 7 min.*

GATHERING ACTIVITY
1. *Show favorite shape*
  - *select shapes from 4 students, try each shape*
  - *class decides order of 4 shapes = 1-2-3-4 and perform pattern*
2. *Pattern combination: Shape 1 + slide right*
  Shape 2 + swing
  Shape 3 + slide left
3. *Show + Share*   *Shape 4 = ending*
	Circle:
	Standing
	
	Scattered
		10-15 min.

RELAXATION *Repeat activities from Lesson one* *"My Body Moves"* *Chapter 10 "Kittens"*	*Circle:* *Sitting* *lying on back*	*5 min*
Evaluation of the lesson: 1. What went well? 2. What can be improved?		

Time Allotment_____

Grade/Age_____

Outline of Lesson Plan One
"How Do I Move"

Number of Students_____

Unit title: *Time* Lesson title: *How Do I Move?* Date:	**Props/Materials:** **Visual Aids:**
Objectives 1. *move body parts fast + slow* 2. *move through space fast + slow* 3. *create a movement pattern*	**Equipment:** *Drum, Gong* *cassette/CD player* **Accompaniment:** *Voice* *percussion, music*

Activities of the Lesson	Formation	Time
WARM UPS 1. *Chant: head, shoulders, knees + toes –* *use different tempos* 2. *Walking: slow to fast, fast to slow*	*Circle:* *Sitting* *Standing* *Scattered*	*5 min.*
MOVEMENT EXPLORATION ACTIVITIES 1. *Shake + freeze body parts* 2. *In place – move body parts fast + slow* 3. *Combine fast + slow movements with levels* 4. *Walk, run at different tempos*	*Circle:* *Standing* *Scattered*	*5-7 min*

GATHERING ACTIVITY
COMBINATIONS: (move, stop, shape)
   1. *Walk, stop, shape (regular tempo)*
   2. *Walk, stop, shape (slow/fast tempos)*
   3. *Run, stop, make shape slowly – repeat*
   4. *Run stop, make shape fast – repeat*
F: Fast: run, stop - FAST moving shape
S: Slow: walk, stop - Slow moving shape
Explore: FSFS – FFSS – SFFS.   *Show + Share*
	Standing
	Scattered
		10-15min

RELAXATION 1. *Stretch to ceiling, bend – touch toes* 2. *"melt"* 3. *Lie quietly, stretch + relax* 4. *Listen to music, eyes closed, relaxed body*	*Standing* *Collapse* *Lying on back*	*5 min.*
Evaluation of the lesson: 1. What went well? 2. What can be improved?		

Outline of Lesson Plan Two
"The Beat Goes On"

	Props/Materials:
Unit title: *Time* Lesson title: *The Beat Goes On* Date:	Visual Aids: *Charts*
Objectives 1. *relate body movements & musical note values* 2. " " *shapes* " " " " 3. *create a pattern*	Equipment: *Drum,* *cassette / CD player* Accompaniment: *Voice,* *percussion, music*

Activities of the Lesson	Formation	Time
WARM UPS 1. *Stretch, bend, "hangover," curl up* 2. *Slow twists side-to-side, rise up + lower down* 3. *Marching - forward, backward* *add - hand clap with march step*	*Circle:* *Sitting* *Standing* *Scattered*	*5 min.*

MOVEMENT EXPLORATION ACTIVITIES
Use Charts
   Sounds - Counting, moving, freezing
   Chart 1 - Hand Clap
   Chart 2 - Feet tap
	Sitting
	group facing
	teacher
		5-7 min.

GATHERING ACTIVITY *Explore rhythmic pattern with words* *at levels of (1) sitting, (2) Standing, (3) moving* *Explore Variation* *Combine pattern with variation (use different* *directions - forward, backward, etc.)* *Show + Share*	*Sit* *Stand* *Scattered*	*10-15 min*
RELAXATION *Stretch arms, legs, alternate R + L* *Breathing ; Close eyes + relax all over* *Slow music - find quiet inner self*	*Lying on back*	*5 min*
Evaluation of the lesson: 1. What went well? 2. What can be improved?		

Outline of Lesson Plan One
"My Place in Space"

Unit title: Space **Lesson title:** My Place in Space **Date:**	**Props/Materials:** Poem "Contrasts in Space" **Visual Aids:** LEAP *(diagram of circle with arrows)* Diagram on board Spots on floor **Equipment:** Drum **Accompaniment:** Voice, percussion
Objectives 1. explore personal space 2. explore general space 3. explore directions + levels 4. Create a movement pattern	

Activities of the Lesson	Formation	Time
WARM UPS 1. Reach out all around - Poem - movement 2. Walk, leap - horizontal space 3. Jump - vertical space 4. Combination: Walk 8, leap 8, jump 4, rest 4	Circle: Sitting Standing Scattered	5 min.
MOVEMENT EXPLORATION ACTIVITIES 1. In place - how many directions can you reach 2. Shapes + directions in space 3. "Branching Out" + levels 4. Walking through space all directions + various levels	Circle Standing Scattered	5-7 min
GATHERING ACTIVITY - FIND YOUR SPOT 1.) 10 counts - go away - return - make shape 2.) 5 counts " " " " " 3.) 15 counts " " " " " Combine above pattern + "branching out" shapes 1.) 5 counts - jump - branch one direction 2.) 10 counts leap - branch two directions 3.) 15 counts walk - branch three directions	Scattered	10-15 min
RELAXATION Gently collapse on the spot Stretch out on back - Lots of space + make Shapes: stretched out, thin, comfortable Relax and breathe	Scattered Lying on back	5 min.
Evaluation of the lesson: 1. What went well? 2. What can be improved?		

Outline of Lesson Plan Two
"Moving Through Space"

Time Allotment_____

Grade/Age_____

Number of Students_____

	Props/Materials:
Unit title: *Space* **Lesson title:** *Moving Through Space* **Date:**	**Visual Aids:** *Draw pathways on the board* 5 1 2
Objectives 1. *explore levels* 2. *explore pathways (curved, straight, angular)* 3. *explore shapes (curved, straight, angular)* 4. *create a movement pattern*	**Equipment:** *Cassette/CD player* **Accompaniment:** *music*

Activities of the Lesson	Formation	Time

WARM UPS *(Select from previous lessons or Ch. 10)*
 Relate lesson to pathways + shapes. Example:
   Stretch - bend (angular, straight)
   Swinging (curved)
   Pathways: slide (straight), walk (angular), run (curved)
	Circle:
	 Sitting
	 Standing
	 Scattered
		5 min.

MOVEMENT EXPLORATION ACTIVITIES
 Levels - low, medium, high - in place
 Pathways in air - arms, legs
 Pathways on floor - walking: straight
                     curved
                     angular
 Combine one locomotor movement with two pathways — Skip: curved, straight
	Standing
	 Lying on back
	 Standing
	 Scattered
		5-7 min

GATHERING ACTIVITY *COMBINATIONS:* *Locomotor Movement* *Pathway* *Shape* *Level* 1. *Run* *curved* *curved* *low* 2. *Slide* *straight* *straight* *high* 3. *Walk* *angular* *angular* *middle* *Show + Share*	*Scattered*	*10-15 min*
RELAXATION *Select from previous lessons or Ch. 10* *Create new activities*		*5 min*
Evaluation of the lesson: 1. What went well? 2. What can be improved?		

Outline of Lesson Plan One
"Force Through Movement"

Unit title: *Force* Lesson title: *Force Through Movement* Date:	Props/Materials: *Poem "A Very Strong Dance"* Visual Aids:
Objectives 1. *explore percussive movements* 2. *improvise - movement pattern combinations* 3. *use poetry to accompany* 4. *students create improvisation*	Equipment: *Drum* *Cassette/CD player* Accompaniment: *voice* *percussion* *music "Mountain King"*

Activities of the Lesson	Formation	Time
WARM UPS *Select nonlocomotor + locomotor movements that relate to the lesson - see other lessons, Ch. 10, or create new activities*		*5 min.*
MOVEMENT EXPLORATION ACTIVITIES 1. *Listen to music "In the Hall of the Mountain King"* 2. *Describe feelings (strong, sharp, forceful)* 3. *Create movements* 4. *Repeat strong movements - various body parts, directions, shapes, levels, tempos* 5. *Poem "A Very Strong Dance" - create movements to poem*	*Circle or group sitting* *Standing* *Scattered*	*5 - 7 min.*
GATHERING ACTIVITY *Improvise movements using music + movement from above to create a piece (new movements can be added, too)* *Ideas for improvs: movements from warm ups, music + poem (movement exploration), and new movements* *Show + Share*	*Scattered*	*10 - 15 min.*
RELAXATION *Contrast - move from forceful or strong to gentle or weak* 1. *Listen to slow music, slowly stretch all body parts* 2. *Slow breathing*	*Circle or scattered* *Lying on back*	*5 min.*
Evaluation of the lesson: 1. What went well? 2. What can be improved?		

Outline of Lesson Plan Two
"Tight and Loose"

Unit title: *Force* **Lesson title:** *Tight and Loose* **Date:**	**Props/Materials:** **Visual Aids:** *Elastic*
Objectives 1. *explore tight movements (tension)* 2. *explore loose movements (relaxed)* 3. *explore tight/loose combinations* 4. *create a new pattern*	**Equipment:** *Drum, Gong cassette/CD player* **Accompaniment:** *Music, voice percussion*

Activities of the Lesson	Formation	Time
WARM UPS *Select nonlocomotor + locomotor movements from previous lessons, Ch. 10, or create new activities that relate to this lesson.* *Shake body parts (loose) Freeze (tight)*		*5 min.*
MOVEMENT EXPLORATION ACTIVITIES 1. *Use elastic to demonstrate tight + loose* 2. *Explore movement tempos (fast + slow)* 3. *Repeat tight/loose movements without demonstration* 4. *Explore tight/loose body parts* 5. *Locomotor movements - tight + loose*	*Circle Sitting* *Standing* *Scattered*	*5-7 min*
GATHERING ACTIVITY *Class creates a pattern combine tight/loose - fast/slow.* Choose: SHAPE, TEMPO, LEVEL, LOCOMOTOR MOVEMENT *Beginning* - (tight or loose shape) : SHAPE # 1 *Middle* {locomotor movement = MOVEMENT {shape - tight or loose = SHAPE #2 {locomotor movement = MOVEMENT *Ending* (tight or loose shape) = SHAPE #3 *show + share*	*Scattered*	*10-15 min.*
RELAXATION (1) *Leg lifts (tight), collapse gently (loose)* (2) *Stretch arms + legs + relax* (3) *Breathe in + tighten (inhale), out-loosen (exhale)* (4) *Relax all body parts*	*Scattered* *Lying on back*	*5 min.*
Evaluation of the lesson: 1. What went well? 2. What can be improved?		

LESSON PLANS
CREATED BY TEACHERS

Since first publishing Adventures in Creative Movement Activities, many requests have been made to create some type of publication that included more lessons; consequently, in this edition,the author has included one of her own lessons (The Penang Lesson), followed by a selection of 28 lessons created and implemented by teachers from preschool through 6th grade.

The 28 lessons appearing in the appendix were copied and edited from the teachers lesson plan outlines by this author for easier reading. During a period of three years, hundreds of Idaho teachers participated in a creative dance project and fulfilled part of the course requirements by designing, teaching, and evaluating lessons taught to their students and submitting their plans to the teaching team for our feedback. The selection was difficult because so many exciting lessons had been created and implemented.

Each one of the 28 lessons provides interesting and innovative ideas that can be adapted to any age group and ability. Feel free to recreate, adapt, or use in tact, any of the lessons that these teachers contributed. This author has added "notes to teachers" and/or "extender ideas" to some of the lessons.

The reader is to assume that the length of the lesson is 25-30 minutes and that each section is approximately the number of minutes suggested in the lesson plan format in Chapter 3. A few of the lessons deviate from the suggested format in order to add necessary details to complete the lesson. Creating your own lesson plan format is perfectly acceptable! A consistent form was attempted to make interpreting the lesson content as quick and easy as possible. A table of contents precedes the lessons to give an overview of the topics that are included.

Special thanks are due to these teachers for contributing a wealth of information concerning the use of creative movement and creative dance with their students. When permission for publishing was requested, every teacher was excited about being a part of this *Adventures* book.

The Penang Lesson mentioned above was "prepared on the spot" by this author while teaching creative dance to preschool and kindertgarten teachers at a workshop in Penang, Malaysia in June 1990. This lesson was created minutes after the first edition of *Adventures* was published, and it was the first of many ideas to be written in the author's book on The Idea Pages. In honor of those teachers in Penang (northern Malaysia) who helped develop this lesson without knowing that it was being created on the spot, the lesson is entitled "The Penang Lesson."

The material in this lesson has become a Movement Exploration Activity leading into the Gathering Activity. The Penang Lesson has been successfully taught to children and adults since 1990. Wrapped in this lesson is the opportunity for learning about another country—geography (where it is), mathematics (how far away it is), and the customs and culture (who the people are, what they do, the holidays they celebrate, and many other details).

The Penang Lesson came as a "flash of insight" as this author was teaching the warm ups and realized that no musical instruments such as a drum, gong, triangle, and a rattle were available to use as accompaniment. (When at home, however, this author uses those instruments to teach this lesson.) When abroad, in Penang, voices became the accompaniment and rarely since that time are instruments used to introduce the qualities of movement because of the successful result that this emergency spawned. The outline of the lesson is included following the instructions.

THE PENANG LESSON

Standing in a circle, movement exploration of each quality was conducted so that the students would understand the differences in energy and time expenditure for each movment. Following this exploration, the lesson culminated in the gathering activity.

The gathering activity incorporated the movement and its quality, vocal sounds, and a counting pattern. The counting pattern used one movement and one sound for the first quality, two movements and two sounds for the second quality, and continued this pattern through to six movements and six sounds. Because the sustained movement was the first to be performed, it received one action and one sound. A cumulative pattern (increasing in force or value by successive additions) was used to build the whole set of six movements: the first movement/sound was performed, the second movement/sound was performed and added to the first action. The best way to interpret a cumulative pattern is to use numbers: 1, 1-2, 1-2-3, 1-2-3-4, 1-2-3-4-5, and 1-2-3-4-5-6. The movement/sound pattern that was built is as follows:

1. **Sustained** Sing the word "G-O-N-G" and simultaneously make one movement until no more sound is heard (because you are out of breath).

2. **Percussive** Make two strong forceful movements (choose body parts, karate movements are a good descriptor) with the loudest voice possible saying "POW - POW" (one POW for each movement).

3. **Staccato** Try three quick, light, sharp movements (flicking kinds of action could use a knee, foot or toe, hand or fingers, nose, tongue) while making a high pitched sound of "EE - EE - EE."

4. **Pendular** Perform four swinging movements (arms swinging from one side to the other and at the lowest point of the arc, knees bend taking the dancer into squat position) while saying "AHHHH" (for each complete swing that is side to side, or back and forth) "AHHHH - AHHHH - AHHHH - AHHHH."

5. **Vibratory** In a standing position, hang the body over so that the arms and shoulders are relaxed and the eyes are looking at the knees. Gently shake all body parts (including the head and face with the jaw relaxed so that even the lips shake) while jogging in place and counting aloud "1 - 2 - 3 - 4 - 5." (No one can see your face, cheeks, and lips shaking .)

6. **Collapse** Moving the body from a high level to a low level as the voice pitch also starts high and finishes low, with a count of "1 - 2 - 3 - 4 - 5 - 6."

Extending the movement pattern can be accomplished by reversing the order and begin with movement/sound six and concluding with movement/sound one.

Another way to"play" with this lesson is to retain the circle formation and divide the class into six groups with each group being assigned (or selecting) one quality to perform. Then have each group perform and complete its movement before the next group begins. Start with group one, the sustained movement/sound, and continue until all groups have performed. Next have group one begin on count 1, group two begin on count 2, and continue until all groups have performed. A round could be created by having each group perform its pattern twice with each group using 6 counts for each pattern or a total of 12 counts.

TEACHER: MARCIA LLOYD
    "The PENANG LESSON" Penang, Malaysia

Time Allotment __30 min__
Grade/Age __Pre-K Teachers__
Number of Students __35__

CREATIVE DANCE - LESSON PLAN OUTLINE

Unit title: *Fundamental Movements* Lesson title: *Qualities of Movement* Date: *June, 1990*	Props/Materials: Visual Aids:

Objectives 1. *learn the qualities* 2. *use vocal sounds to accompany movement* 3. *Create a pattern*	Equipment: Accompaniment:

Activities of the Lesson	Formation	Time
WARM UPS *Stretch + Bend* *Walk, skipping various directions*	*Circle* *Scattered*	*5 min*
MOVEMENT EXPLORATION ACTIVITIES *With no drum, gong, or other instruments* *we used our voices to help learn each one:* *1. Sustained 4. Swing* *2. Percussive 5. Vibrate* *3. Staccato 6. Collapse* *Create a pattern: Cumulation= 1; 1-2; 1-2-3 etc*	*Circle*	*5-7 min*
GATHERING ACTIVITY *1. Sustained (one gong sound with voice) -GONG* *2. Percussive (two "Karate Kicks) POW, POW* *3. Staccato (three quick light movements) "E"E"E" (high voice)* *4. Swinging (swing arms from high to low) and say "AH, AH, AH, AH."* *5. Vibrate (jogging of feet + relax body + face) Count 1-2-3-4-5 will jogging* *6. Collapse (relax to floor) Count from high to low voice*		*15 min*
RELAXATION *1-2-3-4-5-6* *Curl + Breathe* *Stretch*		*5 min*

Evaluation of the lesson: 1. What went well? 2. What can be improved?	

CONTENTS OF LESSON PLANS CREATED BY TEACHERS

LESSON 1: My Heart and What It Does When I Move
Unit Title: My Heart
Teacher: Barbara Chaney
Age group: 3-9 year olds

OBJECTIVES: This experience will identify where the heart is located in the chest cavity and how it sounds before and after movement through an obstacle course call a "Heart Walk"

Equipment:
One (1) listening tent: card table and listening tent cover
5 stethoscopes
1/2 roll freezer wrap paper for obstacle course (directional signs)
2 rolls tape for paper obstacle course
3 chairs
1 balance beam
1 cassette player for musical tape
1 "Mousercize" tape
4 hula hoops
Gauze for stethoscopes
Alcohol for stethoscopes
1 heart poster
1 heart badge per child

STEP 1: The room is set up so that as children come in they enter the "Heart Walk" sign area and sit while they are shown the poster of the heart and then receive their own heart badge which is placed over their own heart so that they will know where to hear their heart sound.

STEP 2: Children proceed to the listening tent where stethoscopes are placed inside the tent and listen to their hearts after they have been sitting and hear it beat.

STEP 3: Children now proceed to the obstacle course as seen in the following diagram of the floor plan.

(Lesson 1, continued)

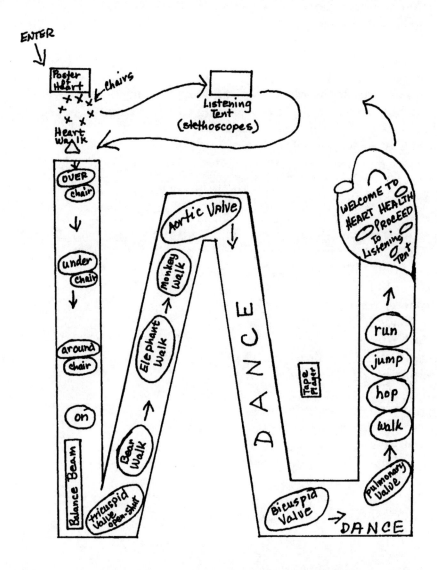

STEP 4: After finishing the obstacle course, children proceed once again to the listening tent and see if they can identify the increased speed of their heart rates.

LESSON 2: A "Beary" Moving Lesson
Unit Title: Concept Words
Teacher: Linda Beamer Shortreed & Carol Ann Nelson
Age group: K-1st Grade

OBJECTIVES
(front-back; big-little; fast-slow)
1. discuss concept words & ways of demonstrating using our bodies
2. discuss concept words as they relate spatially (high-low; near-far)
3. explore levels using concept words
4. look at the world with minds as well as eyes
5. create movement to accompany the book, Going On a Bear Hunt

Materials
Books:
McMillan, Bruce (1986). Becca Backward. Becca Forward. Lothrop Lee & Shepard publishers. (a book of concept pairs)
Hoban, Tana (1972). Push . Pull . Empty . Full. Macmillan Publishers.
Rosen, Michael & Oxenburh, Helen (1989). Going On a Bear Hunt. McElderry Books.

Poster: We Move
Accompaniment: voice, drum, hands
Equipment: tape player/cassette tape

WARM-UPS (circle, standing)
1. stretch high-bend low, reach left-reach right
2. arm bends to side (middle level)
3. arms above head (high level); bend at waist (low level)
4. tortoise-hare run in place (slow-fast)
5. circle game "rig a jig jig" (children create movements to rhythm/tempo of the words)

MOVEMENT EXPLORATION ACTIVITIES
Sit in lines 2x2 facing teacher:
1. ****Brain Gym Activities**: Cook's Hook Up (left/right), Cross Crawls, Elephant (figure 8) high—low
2. Read books—show pictures (Becca; Push-Pull)

Stand in lines:
3. March forward — steady beat—clapping 1-10 March backward — steady beat—snapping 10-1

(Lesson 2, continued)

Partners:
4. Games to develop movements for concept of pairs
    Sing: "Row, row, row, your boat"

    With partner and body movements demonstrate: up/down, push/pull, in/out, thick/thin, front/back, big/little, together/apart, left/right, near/far, over/under, around/through, heavy/light

5. Sing "Itsy, Bitsy Spider" with variations: itsy bitsy—medium, great big—big, teeny weeny—small
    "Jack in the Box," In—low, Out—high

GATHERING ACTIVITY (scattered)

1. Teacher reads Bear Hunt—children think of different ways to use body movements and levels to interpret various segments (teacher observes and comments)

2. One movement for each sequence of the story is selected and the story is told again
    (*story has lots of opportunities for interpretation-different movements and changes in tempo and leads into relaxation activities)

RELAXATION (scattered)

Deep breathing
Brain gym activities: the owl, breathing, head rolls
Quiet relaxing: soft music, lights out

**Dennison, Paul, & Dennison, Gail. (1986). Brain Gym. Simple Activities for Whole Brain Learning. Published by Dennison and Dennison, 616 Viewpoint Circle, Ventura, CA 93003. To order the book, telephone: 1-805-650-3303.

LESSON 3: Machines & Pretending
Unit Title: Creative Movement
Teacher: Debra Lynn Edgett
Age group: 1st Grade

OBJECTIVES
1. to develop imagination
2. to develop group cooperation

Materials
Pictures of different machines

WARM-UPS
1. Read: <u>See Me Run</u> (track formation around the gym) 3 min.
2. Jumping Jacks (own space; 1 min.)
3. Wing stretches (own space; 1 min.)

MOVEMENT EXPLORATION ACTIVITIES (own space)
Pretend:
Children pretend to be popcorn kernels in a pan of oil. Turn up the heat using cues of "hot," "hotter," etc., until the class is "popping." Then pour the popcorn" in a bowl (tumble) and add syrup and popcorn gets sticky and attaches to each other until we are one big popcorn ball. (Repeat)

GATHERING ACTIVITY (groups)
Machine Movement:
Divide into 5 or 6 groups and have children sit in their groups. Each group selects a card that has a picture of a machine on it. Each group will create a movement pattern to show their machine to the class. (Give time for each group to practice their movements before sharing with the class.) When each group shows its "machine movement," the class will guess what the machine is.

RELAXATION
Deep breathing (standing)
Breathe in through the nose and make yourself very tall.
Exhale through the mouth and relax while bending over toward the floor. Repeat.

- -

Ideas for machines:
Toaster, egg beater, mixer, blender, dishwasher, washing machine, dryer, TV, lawnmower, record player, vacuum, hair dryer, bicycle, coffee bean grinder, car, or truck.

LESSON 4: **Let's Visit the Calendar**
Unit Title: Seasons
Teacher: Kaydene Cope
Age Group: K- 1st Grades

OBJECTIVES
1. use of the calendar
2. season awareness
3. develop motor skills—march, toe touches, gallop, skip, balance, hop

Props: Hula hoop, Calendar
Equipment: 1 magic hat, 1 magic hoop
Accompaniment: Music for various seasons—September song, pumpkin, over the river, Santa Claus is Coming, ice skating, Valentine's day, Easter bunny

WARM-UPS (line formation)
Teacher holds the hula hoop and students go through the hoop following directions such as grow and shrink. (The hoop is magic and when the dancers go through they become magic!)

MOVEMENT EXPLORATION ACTIVITIES
Explore locomotor movements of marching, galloping, skipping, hopping.
Explore nonlocomotor movements such as balancing, toe-touching, growing, shrinking
Children go through the magic hoop into "calendar-land"

GATHERING ACTIVITY
1. September - a march and plie (circle)
2. October pumpkin—toe touches and walking (line)
3. November - over the river—gallop (circle)
4. December - Santa coming—skip (line to scatter)
5. January - Ice skating—balance (scatter)
6. February-Valentine—combine nonlocomotor and locomotor movements (scatter)
7. Spring - Bunny—hops (scatter)

RELAXATION
Children go back through the hoop and "home" to stretch out on the floor and "sleep and dream."

LESSON 5: Kindergarten Mouse "Hi To You and Hi To Me!"
Unit Title: Christmas Program Dances
Teacher: Sherry Holman
Age Group: K-2nd Grades

OBJECTIVES
Prepare students for mouse games through: handshakes, slides, movement to music, and learn the dance

Props: colored bracelets (red (R.)/green (L.)); one set for each child, put on proper wrists
Equipment: Records, record player
>   Records:
>   Warm ups —"Mexican Waltz"
>   (Henry "Buzz" Glass—"Rainy Day Records")
>   Mouse Dance —"Hi to You and Hi to Me"
>   (Georgianna Stewart—"Folk Dance Fun")

WARM-UPS   (scattered)
"Mexican Waltz"—reaches, bends, stretches. Move around the room like a mouse and shake hands with others. Keep changing until the teacher blows a whistle.

MOVEMENT EXPLORATION ACTIVITIES (partners)
1. Color-coded hand shakes—Right (red), Left (green), both hands
2. (on tummies on the floor) Mouse-hands under chin—feet gently kicking
3. (standing) create heel/toe sequence and add mouse tail movements
4. slide-play game of mouse trying to run to the side as children practice sliding (sliding 4 with right, then 4 with left)

GATHERING ACTIVITY (partners)
Sequence the dance from the four movement exploration activities and put the whole dance together.
Find school staff to provide the audience for rehearsal (the dance will be presented for parents at a Christmas program)

RELAXATION (scattered)
Closed bottle—pretend you are a mouse caught in a bottle; lie with eyes closed. Feel the walls of the bottle. The bottle is getting smaller/now bigger. Quietly slip out of the bottle and get into the line to return to class as "Quiet as a Mouse!"

LESSON 6: Matching Movement of Body Parts To Beat
Unit Title: Body Parts
Teacher: Jane Wyndham
Age Group: 1st & 2nd Grades

OBJECTIVES
1. participate with others
2. integrate dance into science/health
3. relate movement effectively to accompanying sounds

Props: 9 pieces of yarn = 10 ft. long (for each piece)
Equipment: Triangle, stick, wood block

WARM-UPS (scattered)
Neck: say "No," "Yes," Windshield wiper
Shoulders: say "I don't know," forward, back, rolls
Arms: ins & outs; Waist: forward, back, rolls
Sit on floor: legs apart (little toes down) tap floor with fingertips to left,
    middle, right, reach left, right
Toes: flex, point; Legs together: reach to toes & hold.
Stand, arms hang down.

MOVEMENT EXPLORATION ACTIVITIES (scattered) In each position
teacher asks four questions:
Sitting on floor--How would: 1. eyes blink
Lying on floor --How would: 2. lungs breathe
Standing   --How would: 3. heart beat
                                  4. stomach digest food

moving slowly, then faster

GATHERING ACTIVITY (scattered in groups of 4)
Make a body—1 person = eyes; 1 person = lungs;
    1 person = heart; 1 person = stomach.
Group (or body) moves together holding onto a piece of yarn.

Slow, medium, fast tempos played on wood block or triangle. Bodies move
around the room. When the tempo stops, the body parts move for 4 beats
and then freeze for 8 beats. Include walk, tip-toe, skip, hop; end with slow
movements.

RELAXATION (yarn circles)
Tie the ends of yarn to form smaller circles for each group. Children sit on
opposite sides with yarn on lap. Raise and lower yarn; move yarn to right
and left; move yarn as eye, lung, heart, and stomach. Children lie down on
floor and visualize eyes blinking slowly, lungs breathing slowly, and heart
beating slowly.

LESSON 7: **We Know Letters & Numbers**
Unit Title: Perceptual Motor Activities
Teacher: Sheila Quinton
Age Group: 1st Grade

OBJECTIVES
1. decoding numbers—review A,B,Cs
2. make different levels of movement to form letters
3. explore agility movements

Props: 1 jump rope per set of partners
Equipment: Lummi sticks
Accompaniment: Voice

WARM-UPS (5 lines of 6 students)
1. slide across the room and back
2. skip across the room and back
3. tiptoe across the room, stretch out legs for 8 counts, run back

MOVEMENT EXPLORATION ACTIVITIES (circle sitting)
Sing A,B,C song; count to 26
Standing—each child will take a different letter and form a shape with the
    body (encourage different shapes and levels)

GATHERING ACTIVITY (standing in pairs)
1. Finding the code number: (use 1= "a" 2= "b", etc. 26= "z")
    a. students can count on fingers code number to find out which letter
    of the alphabet it is
    b. teacher (or students) use lummi sticks to beat out code for the class
2. make the letter with the rope
3. play foot games with letter Example: code 5 ="e"—jump and straddle,
    code 10 = "j"—zig-zag jump (ski jump), code 15 = "o"—mud puddle
    jump into & out of

RELAXATION
Sitting in a circle:
1. move neck and shoulders in all possible directions
2. stretch arms, legs, curl upper body
Standing:
3. head, shoulders, knees and toes; move from fast tempo to slow

----
Note to the teacher:
Letters and numbers can be combined to create a variety of shapes and
movement patterns. For example, 5 = "e" could mean 5 skips and then
make an "e" shape; or 5 "e" shapes.

LESSON 8: Rainbow Connection
Unit Title: Colors
Teacher: J. Carpenter
Age Group: Pre K-3rd Grades

OBJECTIVES
1. identify colors of the rainbow
2. explore directions and levels
3. explore large and small groups

Prop: colored streamers (or scarves)
Visual aids: poster of a rainbow
Accompaniment: "The Rainbow Connection" by the Muppets

WARM-UPS (line)
Line up according to rainbow color scheme of clothes children are wearing.
1. stretch body parts ("over the rainbow")
2. explore levels (the highest part to the lowest part of the rainbow)
3. explore directions (forward, backward, sideward)

MOVEMENT EXPLORATION ACTIVITIES (scattered)
Give each child a colored streamer (or scarf) to help further explore levels
and directions. Move streamers forward and backward, overhead, high,
and low.
Call certain colors and give a movement combination: example: red, orange,
yellow move sideways and freeze in a low position; blue, green, purple
move forward and freeze in a high position. (Create other
combinations.)

GATHERING ACTIVITY (groups/scattered)
Create small groups according to color (red group, green group, etc.) Call
the color of a group and give each group a different movement combination
to perform.
Begin with one color and allow that group to perform before allowing
another group to perform. The groups can scatter and dance individually.
Play "Rainbow Connection" having students improvise creating their own
movement combination.

RELAXATION (circle)
With streamers, move slowly in the circle forward, stop and face the center
and stretch a body part toward the center and then outside of the circle.
At the end have small groups (like the red group) place streamers in a row
in the center of the circle until a rainbow is created by the various colored
streamers and all students are sitting in a circle.

LESSON 9: Adventuring with "The Funny Little Woman"
Unit Title: Movement Celebration
Teachers: Melinda Cairl, Mary Empey, Kaye Turner, and Jane
                 Wyndham
Age Group: 1st, 2nd, 6th Grades (This lesson was team taught by 4
                 teachers with a total of 66 students in the multipurpose room
                 at an elementary school.)

OBJECTIVES
1. students will relate movement effectively to literature
2. students will give form to creative impulses
3. students will perform in front of peers

Visual Aids: Poster of body positions/body parts
Equipment: **Video camera, VCR tape, book—"The Funny Little
   Woman," by Arlene Mosel.
Accompaniment: sound system for microphone, cassette player, music
   tape: Melodies of Japan.

WARM-UPS (scattered) (led by Mary and Kaye)
Sitting: neck: side-to-side, down and up; shoulders: up, down, rolling
shoulders and elbows; legs: spread—bend and reach and slowly up.
Standing: quadriceps stretch, ankle rotations, arms stretch/bend.

MOVEMENT EXPLORATION ACTIVITIES (scattered)
(led by Mary and Kaye)
1. explore movements that look like real-life actions (pantomime)
2. demonstrate each story action element and locations for story action
3. encourage students to create own actions

GATHERING ACTIVITY (MAIN EVENT) (scattered)
(led by Melinda Cairl, story read by Kaye Turner)
1. Class is separated into 2 groups. Groups will alternate as performers
    and audience.
2. Storyteller reads story as students follow the leader to locations and
    through actions of the story.
3. Change groups and repeat.

RELAXATION (scattered, facing posters) (led by Jane Wyndham) Music
played for accompaniment.

Body-parts posters depicting various parts in a variety of positions. Children
look at posters and try the different positions. **Later students were shown
the videotape of their dancing.

LESSON 10: **Animal Movements**
Unit Title: Imagery
Teacher: Rose Marie Adams
Age Group: 2nd Grade

OBJECTIVES
1. explore ways different animals move
2. move at different tempos and levels
3. create a movement pattern

Visual aids: Pictures of animals
Equipment: Drum
Accompaniment: Voice and drum

WARM-UPS (standing, scattered)
1. Head, shoulders, knees, & toes
2. stretch & bend; tight & loose
3. swing and sway
4. leap and hop

MOVEMENT EXPLORATION ACTIVITIES Sit—group, facing teacher:
Show animal pictures; identify body parts, body movements, shapes, levels.
Scattered: Children role-play each animal:
>   1. horse galloping across a meadow and slowing to walk
>   2. elephant lumbering along
>   3. bunny hopping and trying to hide
>   4. eagle soaring at different levels and speed
>   5. lion stalking prey

GATHERING ACTIVITY (scattered)
Pick a favorite animal (need not be from above) and establish a movement
pattern at different tempos, shapes, levels
>   Move quickly forward 8 counts
>   Move slowly in another direction 8 counts
>   Make a shape and freeze for 4 counts

Show and share. (Children may do a particular animal movement pattern
alone or in small groups.)

RELAXATION (scattered, lying on back)
1. Leg lifts (tighten), release to floor (loosen)
2. Stretch arms and legs and relax
3. Breathe in and tighten, Breathe out and loosen
4. Relax all body parts beginning with head and work down to toes

LESSON 11: **How Sound Travels**
Unit Title: Sound
Teacher: Susan Hutchinson
Age Group: 2nd Grade

"In advance of this lesson, I created eight placards with the words, *vibration, eardrum, hammer, anvil, stirrup, cochlea, nerves, and brain,* written one per card. The cards were hung from strings so that each child could hang one around his neck.

Next, eight children were chosen to represent each one of the words on the cards. Before we got into any movement, we discussed the word 'vibration' and the various possibilities for movement when it was that child's turn to vibrate.

The activity began by having someone in the room make a sound. It was 'vibration's' job to vibrate through the air until it came in contact with the eardrum which then began to vibrate against the hammer, and you can see the natural progression. Each child got to vibrate up against the next part until the sound reached the brain."

OBJECTIVES
1. to identify parts of the ear
2. to describe the movement of sound
3. to experience creative movement

Visual aids: Cards with parts of the ear on them
Accompaniment: Voice

WARM-UPS (lines facing teacher)
1. toe taps
2. knee lifts
3. twists & shapes
4 elbow curls

MOVEMENT EXPLORATION ACTIVITIES (circle)
1. Show pictures and identify parts of the ear
2 Choose students to represents (1) vibrate, (2) ear drum, (3) hammer, (4) anvil, (5) stirrup, (6) cochlea, (7) nerves, (8) brain
3. Questions to create movement: How many ways can the body vibrate to show the movement of sound?

GATHERING ACTIVITY (scattered)
1. Divide students into groups of 8
2. Allow groups to work to create their representation of sound moving through the ear
3. Group presentations of sound

(Lesson 11, continued)

RELAXATION (scattered)
1. Standing, stretch high and breathe deeply; curl down and exhale. Repeat.
2. Head rolls—side, forward, side
3. Sit down, bend and stretch (toe touching, etc.)
4. Lying flat on back, do relaxation talk

Other ideas to extend this lesson could be to explore the shapes of the different parts of the ear and what kinds of movements these parts could make. What kinds of locomotor movements could these parts make? Explore sounds heard by the ear. What kind of movements can be made when you can barely hear the sound? when the sound is very loud, shrill, deep, etc.?

LESSON 12: Clocks
Unit Title: Use of Time
Teacher: Deanna Hovey
Age Group: 2nd Grade

OBJECTIVES
1. concept of hour hand moves slow; minute hand moves fast
2. learn to position self as hour or minute hand
3. create a "moving clock"

Visual aids: Cards with numbers 1-12
Equipment: Clock with an alarm

WARM-UPS (scattered)
What does a clock say? (Tick Tock).
Show tick tock with head, also other body parts
How do clock hands move? Show circular movements with various body parts.

MOVEMENT EXPLORATION ACTIVITIES (scattered)
1. Walk the way you do when you are rushed for time
2. Walk as if you don't want to get some place
3. Walk forward, backward, and sideways. Change directions when you hear the alarm ring

GATHERING ACTIVITY (clock formation, circles)
(2 clock formations) Divide into 2 groups of 14 each. If smaller groups make 12, 3, 6, and 9 on clock) Have children hold numbers and position themselves around the circle like clock numbers. Two children are hands. Teacher gives a time, the two students lie on the floor as clock hands at the proper numbers. Change "hands" and numbers until all have had turns.

RELAXATION (scattered)
Lie down, close eyes. Guess how long a minute is. Raise your hand when you think a minute is up.

Ideas to extend the clock lesson could be to use each wall of the room as a time (12, 3, 6, 9) and have students use a certain locomotor movement to travel to the "12:00, 3:00, 6:00, 9:00" wall(s). Upon arrival at the "hour wall" students could create a shape or shapes for as many counts as the number of the wall. If students travel to the "6:00 wall" they could stop and make 6 shapes at different levels. Diagonal corners could be used for the half hour location and a different movement task could be created for this corner. Ask the students what kinds of movements could be performed at various "clock" locations in the room.
Another could be to create a shape at the numbered wall for 12, 9, 6, or 3 seconds. The student could use the count of "one-on thousand, two-one thousand, etc." for the time to hold the shape for the number of seconds required.

LESSON 13: Dinosaur Movement
Unit Title: Prehistoric Animals
Teacher: Deanna Hovey
Age group: 2nd Grade

OBJECTIVES
1. explore 3 levels of space: high, medium, low
2. movement around the room at different speeds

Props: Drum
Visual aids: Pictures of dinosaurs
Accompaniment: Drum

WARM-UPS (scattered)
Dinosaurs waking up. In area where students are not touching others, "wake up" isolated parts and move as dinosaur might have—head, shoulders, arms, waist, legs, feet

MOVEMENT EXPLORATION ACTIVITIES (scattered)
All make:

> HIGH shapes = tyrannosaurus
> MEDIUM height-long shape = Apatosaurus
> LOW small shape = Compsognathus

1. On drum beat change shapes (take each level one at a time)
2. In time to the beat, pick shape and move as slowly or quickly as the particular dinosaur

GATHERING ACTIVITY (end of gym to other end of gym)
Game—Tar Pit. Divide class in thirds: 1/3 of class to be tyrannosaurus, 1/3 Apatosaurus, 1/3 Compsognathus.
When name is called, students must run from one end of the gym to the other, leaping over area between tape (tar pit). If foot lands in area, they are caught. Proceed until many have landed in tar pit. (Others may escape.)

RELAXATION (floor, line)
"Caught" dinosaurs drink at LaBrea Tar Pits and are stuck and sink. (floor)
Those dinosaurs not caught turn into Paleontologists who discover the bones of the others who were caught and take them carefully to the museum. (line)

Note to teachers: Remember: A dinosaur can become a "Dansosaurus!"
Also other dinosaurs can be explored.

LESSON 14: The Very Busy Spider
Unit Title: Story Movement
Teacher: Janet Filpi
Age group: 2nd Grade

OBJECTIVES
1. listening
2. exploring animal movement through different body shapes

Visual aids: Photos of a spider and its parts
                 Book: The Very Busy Spider by Eric Carle
Accompaniment: Voice

WARM-UPS (circle standing, scattered)
Stretching arms—make circles, twist waists, roll neck, bends at waist, floor scooting

MOVEMENT EXPLORATION ACTIVITIES (sitting scattered; scattered moving high/low)
Introduce story title for book, The Very Busy Spider. Discuss spider parts
    (8 legs, etc.).
Explore moving like a spider.
Explore moving like other animals—horse, cow eating grass, sheep running
    in meadow, etc.

GATHERING ACTIVITY (use whole gym, scattered)
Stay close enough to hear story—moving without talking.

Teacher reads story and class creates movements of animals in the story—
moving around the room

RELAXATION (scattered, but sitting close to teacher)
Teacher tells them to move like a spider after spinning a web all day. Sit,
legs spread. Inch fingers along legs crawling like a spider to stretch. Shake
out legs. Then pretend to nap or rest.

EVALUATION (The teacher reported the results of this lesson)
"Great—they loved it! Listening was at a maximum. Recall of the story
at a later time was almost 100%. They used imaginations to create many
different shapes and movements for each story character. Fun!"

LESSON 15: The Very Busy Spider (a different lesson)
Unit Title: Reading is Movin' Our Way (Body)
Teacher: Teresa Bala
Age group: 2nd Grade

OBJECTIVES
1. identify body parts
2. listen and comprehend story
3. explore different levels
4. explore locomotor skills by using "verbs" in story

Props/Materials: Stuffed snake and book, <u>The Very Busy Spider</u>
Equipment: whistle
Accompaniment: voice

WARM-UPS Stitting with legs crossed:
1. Boa Constrictor (song)
2. neck circles—4 counts—slow
3. arms circles—4-4 counts each way
Also could include stretching out legs by being little spiders and crawling finger tips on legs down to toes.
Standing and scattered:
4. berry pickers—4-4 counts
5. jog (not run) and then freeze

MOVEMENT EXPLORATION ACTIVITIES
(sitting—group facing teacher)
Explain to children they will be "acting out" the story by listening for certain clues (example: spider spins). (Scattered in half of the gym) Show me: wind <u>blowing,</u> spider <u>spinning</u>, <u>riding</u> a horse, <u>running</u> in meadow, <u>jumping</u> on rocks, <u>rolling</u> in mud, etc.
When you hear the whistle blow, you will listen to the next page.

GATHERING ACTIVITY (scattered, use the whole gym)
Read story and have kids create movement to each page. Teacher may participate. ("I enjoyed watching.")

RELAXATION (scattered, lie down on backs)
Explain that all the "spiders" are tired from their busy day and need to relax. Have them cross arms over chest, knees bent, and slow down their breathing by talking them into being quiet.

EVALUATION The teacher stated: "The children loved this and begged to do it again—which we did! One child said 'I never knew you could do neat things with books!' Great lesson."

LESSON 16: Let's Push Some Space Around
Unit Title: Space Awareness/Body Awareness
Teacher: Melinda Cairl
Age group: 2nd Grade

OBJECTIVES Each child will:
1. develop sense of "space"
2. explore physical movement
3. explore rhythmic movement moving "space"
4. create movement representation of an object

Equipment: Book: Theater Games for the Classroom by Viola Spolin
                Boundary markers
Accompaniment: Music with strong rhythms of various kinds and a record
    player

WARM-UPS (scattered, partners, standing)
Do a series of nonlocomotor and locomotor warm ups based on pushing
and pulling space (or air) around us.
(Review space exercises, group & partners)

MOVEMENT EXPLORATION ACTIVITIES (within confines of
boundary and scattered)
Play a few minutes of explosion tag (p. 25)
Present game of slow motion/Freeze Tag
    — set boundaries, 2 taggers if needed
    — everyone runs and breathes in slow motion
    — once "It" tags another, then old "It" freezes (p. 32)

GATHERING ACTIVITY (scattered in playing area)
Rhythmic Movement.
Select coaches. Group is divided as audience and players.
Coach calls out objects and players move in "spirit" with that object.
Rotate coaches, audience, players.
Play music as players find their rhythm
Suggested objects: washing machine, dryer, sprinkler, TV, circus artists,
etc. (p. 33)

RELAXATION (scattered, seated)
Feeling Self with Self (p. 37)
Coach guides players — keep your eyes opened! Now, feel your feet in
your socks! Feel your socks on your feet! etc.

LESSON 17: The Turtles & The Hares
Unit Title: The Body
Teacher: Teresa Bala
Age group: 2nd Grade

OBJECTIVES
1. explore locomotor skills
2. demonstrate understanding of relay race
3. identify body parts

Props/Materials: 4 colored squares numbered 1 thru 4
Visual aids: Pictures of turtles/hares
Equipment: whistle, cassette tape & player, drum
Accompaniment: The Lone Ranger music, voice, percussion

WARM-UPS
Circle—standing and holding hands
1. March in place-16 counts-knees high
2. "Noble Duke of York"
Sitting:
3. Legs apart-twist-snap (4 counts)
4. Legs apart-alternate stretching over legs (4 counts)

MOVEMENT EXPLORATION ACTIVITIES
Sitting facing teacher, use half of gym:
Call for different volunteers to demonstrate: walk, run, hop, skip, jump, gallop, leap, slide, roll
Scattered formation using whole gym:
Have entire class demonstrate the locomotor movements
Listen for drum beat for new directions

GATHERING ACTIVITY
Standing:
Have children line up in one row (lunch line order). Number off 1 thru 4. Show students the squares and have them line up behind the squares.
Standing in lines (one person behind another):
Explain the concept of a relay race. Students will run (or some other locomotor movement) to a designated line (middle line of the gym) and return to the end of their line. The teacher participates so that there is a "turtle." Children will listen to locomotor skill called for each group.

(Lesson 17, continued)

RELAXATION (circle standing; circle sitting)
1. Breathe-rag doll curl downs — 3 times
2. Sit up straight-deep breathing — 3 times
3. Bend over and grab ankles — 3 times (4 counts each time)
4. Shake out legs; shake out arms
5. Stand up and walk like Frankenstein to the door

EVALUATION "The children had a ball. They were extremely tickled that I would participate. They need more practice with leaping unlike a frog. Will do this again. We were all laughing and having fun. Note: I was surprised at the kids when they didn't know what sitting up straight meant!"

LESSON 18: Minute Men & Paul Revere
Unit Title: Paul Revere
Teacher: Sherry Holman
Age group: 3rd Grade

OBJECTIVES
1. creative play
2. learn about Minute Men
3. learn about Paul Revere and the Ride
4. develop galloping skills
5. develop vocabulary words

Visual aids: Book about Paul Revere and the Minute Men
Equipment: Mats, hockey sticks
Accompaniment: voice

WARM-UPS (scattered)
Divide into groups of three: mother, dad, child who are sleeping (on mat) with "gun" (hockey sticks) nearby. Dads practice getting up quickly pretending to dress (drill for 10 seconds);
Mothers/Children help—Dressed in One Minute.
Assign: who will give gun, boots, powder purse, hats, coats to the men

MOVEMENT EXPLORATION ACTIVITIES (scattered)
Explore differences between
     British Rebels way of fighting—straight lines and open formation
     Colonists—hide behind rocks, trees; crawl on stomach; shoot from knees
     Rebels—some die, run, surrender (you choose); switch sides

GATHERING ACTIVITY (scattered)
Divide into 2 teams.
     #1 team = use mats as boats and sticks as oars. Watching lanterns,
          they say as they watch and then rowing—"one if by land,"
          "two if by sea"
     #2 team = horse rider (use hockey stick). Pretend to alert Minute Men-
          "The Redcoats are coming," and gallop all around the room.
Switch places to allow everyone to be part of both team #1 and #2.

RELAXATION (scattered)
"Minute Men" go back to mats and rest after a long evening and day. Repeat and look at "The Old North Tower" saying softly "one if land; two if by sea."

EVALUATION The teacher stated: "The most fun unit. The half hour flew by. A lot of information was learned."

LESSON 19: I Can Be A Skyscraper, A Hotel, A Home
Unit Title: Levels—Skyscrapers, Hotels, Home
Teacher: Ruthanne Jenkins
Age group: 3rd Grade

OBJECTIVES
1. to use body like a skyscraper, hotel, house
2. explore levels of these three buildings
3. create a body movement pattern

Visual aids: Pictures of skyscraper, hotel, home
Accompaniment: Voice, drum

WARM-UPS (straight line, 4 lines)
1. sky reaches (skyscraper)
2. side-to-side extensions (hotel)
3. sit ups (home)

MOVEMENT EXPLORATION ACTIVITIES (scattered)
Show pictures of skyscrapers, hotels, homes. Discuss lines, show different positions at each level.

Skyscrapers - high arm movements
Hotels - arms down to medium position
Homes - arms in low position

Read Poem "Skyscrapers" and have students interpret words with movements

GATHERING ACTIVITY (scattered)
Use drum to help count movement pattern: (body, body parts move to each level)

10 counts	low homes
10 counts	medium hotels
10 counts	high skyscrapers
10 counts	medium hotels
10 counts	low homes

RELAXATION (sitting in a circle)
Shake hands, shake feet
Shake arms, shake legs
Gently shake head, shake whole body
Lie on back and relax.

Note to teachers: For a variation: have students choose one level (skyscraper, hotel, home) and create a movement pattern that would indicate the building). There should be different levels being performed at the same

(Lesson 19, continued)

time.   A lesson extender could be to ask children to select other types of structures and create movement patterns that illustrate the shape, level, and activities that would occur with a teepee, a cave dwelling, a ski lodge, a farm house, etc. A search for more poetry pertaining to buildings could be conducted and use the resulting stimuli for creating more "building dances."

LESSON 20: Mirandy and Brother Wind (African Folk Tale)
Unit Title: African Folk Tales
Teacher: Jan Hamilton
Age group: 3rd Grade

OBJECTIVES

use creative movements to portray characters of "Brother Wind" and Mirandy

Props/Materials: Scarves; Book—Mirandy and Brother Wind
Accompaniment: Voice

WARM-UPS (scattered)

1. practice swinging, twirling, whirling motions
2. practice twirling scarves (various levels, tempos)
3. ready story (2 times)

MOVEMENT EXPLORATION ACTIVITIES (scattered)

1. teach cake walk dance
2. explore movement for Brother Wind

GATHERING ACTIVITY (1/2 of class at a time; audience/performers)

Select Brother Wind and Mirandy.
Read story aloud. Stop and Brother Wind moves with scarves (alone) and Mirandy moves twirling swinging, dancing (alone).
Rest of the class moves as wind.
Repeat with the other 1/2 of the class
Have whole class perform the Cake Walk

RELAXATION (circle)

All relax, hunch down as Brother Wind comes by and leaves a quiet, peaceful swaying group. Have the group stretch and bend gently.

Note: for information about the Cake Walk begin with Let's Dance. Social, Ballroom & Folk Dancing by Peter Buckman (1978), pp. 160-4; 267.

McKissack, Patricia. (1988). Mirandy and Brother Wind. NY: Knopf.

LESSON 21: Baseball Dance
Unit Title: Sport Dances
Teacher: Alice Bradford
Age group: 3rd & 4th Grades

OBJECTIVES
design a dance using movements from baseball

Equipment: record player
Accompaniment: record "Movin'" (by Hap Palmer)

WARM-UPS (scattered)
1. Pitch - slow, fast, high, low
2. Bat - change pathway, add a turn
3. Running - change direction, large & small steps
4. Catching - various levels, freeze

MOVEMENT EXPLORATION ACTIVITIES (scattered)
Explore ways of combining and sequencing movements.
Explore ways of ending the "game" including winning, and losing

GATHERING ACTIVITY (scattered)
Sequence the 4 movements to form an individual dance.
End the dance by jumping up and down, hugging, or shaking hands to express the excitement of winning a game. (make every child a winner!)
Divide class into fourths; have 1/4 perform while others watch. Repeat until everyone has had a chance to perform.

RELAXATION (large circle)
Listen to "Gentle Sea" (on the "Movin'" record) and move according to the way the music makes you feel.

Note: "Take Me Out To The Ball Game" could be another song to use for accompaniment. Other sports could be volleyball, basketball, soccer, skating, skiing, gymnastics, and skateboarding.

LESSON 22: Chinese Zodiac Signs
Unit Title: Chinese Movement Celebration
Teacher: Mary Empey
Age group: 4th & 5th Grades

OBJECTIVES
1. identify and learn about your individual sign
2. give creative form and movement to the sign
3. perform in front of peers

Props: Chinese costume
Equipment: Handouts of Chinese Zodiac Signs
Accompaniment: Oriental music

WARM-UPS (scattered)
1. head, shoulders, knees, and toes
2. stretch & bend
3. twist torso
4. shake out entire body

MOVEMENT EXPLORATION ACTIVITIES (large group, then break into smaller groups)
1. Introduce and explain handout on Chinese signs
2. Explore movements that look like signs
3. Divide into groups to create and show individual signs

GATHERING ACTIVITY (in groups of 4)
Working in groups of 4, demonstrate creative movement pattern of your sign.
Show and Share.
Have each group show its "sign."
(As an extender to the lesson, two signs could be combined to explore how different signs may or may not complement each other.)

RELAXATION (scattered)
1. breathe, curl down and up
2. neck curls
3. deep breathing—let in and let out

Note: This lesson could be combined with an art lesson having students create their own signs (either using the suggested sign or creating a new sign) by drawing, painting, paper mache, making a mural, or using some other medium to create a piece of visual art. This lesson could be combined with world geography, social science, music, or a lesson about foods of the Chinese culture (rice, noodles, tea, fortune cookies, etc.)

LESSON 23: How Your Body Interprets
Unit Title: Interpreting Words
Teacher: Nancy McCoy
Age group: 5th & 6th Grades

OBJECTIVES
1. help children learn to express their feelings with words
2. express words with motion and emotion
3. learn vocabulary

Props/Materials: Vocabulary Words
Visual aids: Social Studies Book
Equipment: Book & Vocabulary sheets

WARM-UPS (classroom beside desks)
1. students need to have looked up and written out definitions of words
2. head and neck rotations
3. stretch and bend

MOVEMENT EXPLORATION ACTIVITIES (beside desks)
1. As a class, decide on a movement that fits each word
2. Practice words and movements
3. Create movements for the definition of each word

GATHERING ACTIVITY (beside desks)
1. Teacher calls off vocabulary words
2. Students show movement and give the definition
3. Students work in pairs alternating giving each other words and definitions and the movement pattern for each word

Vocabulary: SOUTHERNERS, NORTHERNERS, SLAVES, ABOLITIONIST, UNDERGROUND RAILROAD, SECEDE, FUGITIVE SLAVE LAWS, COMPROMISE, UNION, CONFEDERATE

RELAXATION (by desk)
1. deep breathing
2. raggedy Anne's & Andy's
3. more deep breathing

EVALUATION The Teacher commented: "Excellent way for children to learn vocabulary. I'm sure they'll never forget what an Abolitionist believed!"

LESSON 24: What Are We?
Unit Title: Exploring Shapes
Teacher: Nancy McCoy
Age group: 5th & 6th Grades

OBJECTIVES
1. exploring space and various shapes
2. conditioning
3. physical fitness

Visual aids: Pictures of animals (one for each student)
Equipment: Drum, Boombox
Accompaniment: Music with upbeat tempo

WARM-UPS (scattered)
1. reach high, low, center 10 times
2. stretch and make a "C"
3. look high, low behind

MOVEMENT EXPLORATION ACTIVITIES (scattered)
Give students animal pictures; students create a movement that reminds
them of the animal in the picture. (If time permits, have students trade
pictures and create another "animal movement.") Explore a movement game
of shaping statues —partners share in being a statue and a creator placing
the statue in certain shapes by gently moving the limbs, torso, head, etc.

GATHERING ACTIVITY
Divide students into 4 groups.
Ask each group to select a sport that could include high, low, and touching
movements.
Send each group to a corner of the gym to complete the assignment of
creating its own theme, motion, and movement.
Show and Share

RELAXATION (scattered)
1. Lie on the floor and stretch out with limbs
2. Curl up like a ball

EVALUATION: "WOW! My students did a wonderful job. My boys
really got into the shapes and statues. They had no problem touching each
other!"

Note: Another idea is to have students choose a letter, then create a list of
animals (or objects) that begin with that letter and create shapes, build a
movement pattern, and include sounds of the animal. Example: the letter
"C:" cat, canary, crane, crow, cow, cockroach, "critter!" (Of course the
"critter" could be anything.)

LESSON 25: The Teacher From The Black Lagoon
Unit Title: Creative Movement in the Curriculum
Teacher: Sharel Judy
Age group: 5th Grade

OBJECTIVES
1. learn to express themselves with body movements
2. use creative movements to go with a story

Equipment: Book—The Teacher From The Black Lagoon
Accompaniment: voice, drum

WARM-UPS (scattered)
Free movement around the gym using locomotor and axial movements in relation to space, time, force and energy

MOVEMENT EXPLORATION ACTIVITIES (scattered)
Free expression with creative movement while listening to the story
Rules: 1. Cannot talk
       2. Cannot touch anyone else

GATHERING ACTIVITY (sitting in semi-circle)
Review some of the movements students used for descriptions in the story (Example: "In slithers Mrs. Green, she's really green! She has a tail. She scratches her name on the blackboard—with her claws.")

RELAXATION (scattered)
Have students lie on floor totally relaxed

EVALUATION
"I was totally amazed at how freely they acted out this story. They loved it. They came up with some very clever actions. There were some who just copied other students' actions, but most tried to be original. When we finished the story they were eager to do another one."

Thaler, Mike. (1989). The Teacher From the Black Lagoon.
New York, NY: Scholastic, Inc.

LESSON 26: Build a Tree
Unit Title: Sensory Science
Teacher: Gretchen Massman
Age group: 5th Grade

OBJECTIVES
1. to identify the parts of a growing tree
2. to understand the importance of each part to the survival of the tree
3. to create movement and sound to represent the trees life processes

Visual aids: Poster: How a Tree Grows
Accompaniment: voices

WARM-UPS (circle, sitting)
Experiment with various sounds for tree parts such as:
1. heartwood—thump, thump
2. roots - sucking sound
3. xylum - low to high
4. cambium growth rings - pop sound
5. phloem - high to low
6. bark protection - hummm

MOVEMENT EXPLORATION ACTIVITIES (circle, standing)
Warm ups 1-6 put a movement to each function of the tree

(Can choose volunteers to model movements for group, or just let the group create individual movements)

GATHERING ACTIVITY (circle)
Sound and movement for 1-6
1. heartwood - thump, thump—turning
2. roots - sucking sound—pulling up
3. xylum - low to high—rise up
4. cambium growth rings - pop sound—jump
5. phloem - high to low—sink down
6. bark protection - hummm—form barrier

Extension: Spring—speed up; Bugs invade (buzzz)

RELAXATION (circle)
Winter - all activity slows down in the tree until almost stopped— dormant.

LESSON 27: West Indies Map Study

Unit Title: Social studies
Teacher: Carole Schlapia
Age group: 6th Grade Resource Room

OBJECTIVES

1. identify different countries
2. name capitals of these countries
3. create a movement pattern

Visual aids: Map of the West Indies
Equipment: Blackboard with map drawn

WARM-UPS (standing)

1. circle with head
2. snap fingers
3. lift shoulders
4. walk, skip in a variety of directions

MOVEMENT EXPLORATION ACTIVITIES (circle; scattered)

Look at map and identify country and capital. Ask students to express (through movement) a way to get to a place to swim, a way to swim, float, fly, or hop from one island to another

GATHERING ACTIVITY (circle, sitting)

Deep breathing - 4 counts
Picture a place on your mental screen - 4 counts
Stretch in the direction of a country on the map - 4 counts
Add: a snap, skip, swim, or other movements appropriate to remembering countries and capitals and traveling to these places

RELAXATION (circle, standing)

1. breathe, curl down, up
2. neck circles
3. tight and loose

LESSON 28: Events in Nature
Unit Title: Dancing With Mother Nature
Teacher: Kristin Ehler
Age group: Any grade level

OBJECTIVES
1. explore levels and directions
2. name and explore events in nature
3. create movement patterns

Visual aids: Pictures of events in nature
Equipment: cassette player/tape of nature sounds
Accompaniment: music, voice

WARM-UPS (circle—earth)
1. Sunrise
2. Tree in the wind (swing)
3. Rain (run in place)
4. Snow (start high and collapse slowly)
5. Hail (bouncing/stomping in place)

MOVEMENT EXPLORATION ACTIVITIES (scattered, in place)
Explore movements of event:

1. wind
2. ice (freeze)
3. tornado
4. volcano
5. earthquake
6. hail storm
7. rain
8. hurricane

GATHERING ACTIVITY (scattered, using locomotor movements)
Explore movements in nature using directions and levels (individually)
   Directions—forward, backward, sideways, diagonally
   Levels—high, medium, low
The pattern will be a freeze, movement, freeze pattern. Example:
   Volcano-low to high—Freeze
   Earthquake-high or low, moving forward/sideways—Freeze
   Tornado-high or low, moving backwards/diagonally—Freeze
   Individual choice-high or low, choice of direction—Freeze

RELAXATION (circle)
1. Sunset - collapse to sitting
2. Turning body parts - Earth rotating
3 Sway body parts - leaf fluttering on the breeze
4. Rain—bend knees and have feet tap
5. Clouds - lying down

Note: Extend the lesson by grouping students according to an event and have each group create a movement pattern for its event. Present each event. Merge two events for interesting choreographic experiences.

EXTRA LESSON PLAN FORMS

CREATIVE DANCE - LESSON PLAN OUTLINE

Unit title: Lesson title: Date:	Props/Materials: Visual Aids:
Objectives	Equipment: Accompaniment:

Activities of the Lesson	Formation	Time
WARM-UPS		
MOVEMENT EXPLORATION ACTIVITIES		
GATHERING ACTIVITY		
RELAXATION		
Evaluation of the lesson: 1. What went well? 2. What can be improved?		

CREATIVE DANCE - LESSON PLAN OUTLINE

Unit title: *Lesson title:* *Date:*	*Props/Materials:* *Visual Aids:*
Objectives	*Equipment:* *Accompaniment:*

Activities of the Lesson	Formation	Time
WARM-UPS		
MOVEMENT EXPLORATION ACTIVITIES		
GATHERING ACTIVITY		
RELAXATION		
Evaluation of the lesson: 1. What went well? 2. What can be improved?		

CREATIVE DANCE - LESSON PLAN OUTLINE

Unit title: Lesson title: Date:	Props/Materials: Visual Aids:
Objectives	Equipment: Accompaniment:

Activities of the Lesson	Formation	Time
WARM-UPS		
MOVEMENT EXPLORATION ACTIVITIES		
GATHERING ACTIVITY		
RELAXATION		
Evaluation of the lesson: 1. What went well? 2. What can be improved?		

CREATIVE DANCE - LESSON PLAN OUTLINE

Unit title: Lesson title: Date:	Props/Materials: Visual Aids:
Objectives	Equipment: Accompaniment:

Activities of the Lesson	Formation	Time
WARM-UPS		
MOVEMENT EXPLORATION ACTIVITIES		
GATHERING ACTIVITY		
RELAXATION		
Evaluation of the lesson: 1. What went well? 2. What can be improved?		

CREATIVE DANCE - LESSON PLAN OUTLINE

Unit title: Lesson title: Date:		Props/Materials: Visual Aids:	
Objectives		Equipment: Accompaniment:	
Activities of the Lesson		**Formation**	**Time**
WARM-UPS			
MOVEMENT EXPLORATION ACTIVITIES			
GATHERING ACTIVITY			
RELAXATION			
Evaluation of the lesson: 1. What went well? 2. What can be improved?			

CREATIVE DANCE - LESSON PLAN OUTLINE

Unit title: *Lesson title:* *Date:* *Objectives*	*Props/Materials:* *Visual Aids:* *Equipment:* *Accompaniment:*	
Activities of the Lesson	**Formation**	**Time**
WARM-UPS		
MOVEMENT EXPLORATION ACTIVITIES		
GATHERING ACTIVITY		
RELAXATION		
Evaluation of the lesson: 1. What went well? 2. What can be improved?		

INDEX

Levels, 17, 103
Locomotor movements 18, 164

M

Maryland Council for Dance, 238
Mayfield Publishing Company, 238
Minnesota Center for Arts Education, 238
Movement:
      collapse, 126, 271
      locomotor, 18, 164
      nonlocomotor, 18, 164
      pendular, 125, 271
      percussive, 125
      staccato, 125, 271
      sustained, 125, 271
      swinging, 164
      swaying, 164
      vibratory, 126, 271
Movement exploration, 26
Movement exploration activities:
      The Body
            lesson one, 55-57
            lesson two, 68
            Body Wheels, 75
            body words, 74
      Time:
            lesson one, 83-84
            lesson two, 89-92
            time words, 97
      Space:
            lesson one, 108-110
            lesson two, 115-116
            space words, 120
      Force
            lesson one, 126-128
            lesson two, 131-133
            force words, 137
Multicultural ideas, 158
Music sources, 238
Musical note values, 90

N

National Association for the Education of Young Children, 237
National Dance Association, 237

National Standards for Dance, 227-230
Nonlocomotor movements 18, 164
Nursery rhymes, 175-179

O

Objectives
      creative movement, 8
      lesson plan format, 26
      lessons created by teachers, 274-306
      My Body, 47, 64
      Time, 82, 88
      Space,106, 115
      Force, 126, 131
      The Penang Lesson, 271
Organizations promoting dance, 237-238

P

Pathways, 17, 104, 115-121
Pendular movement, 125
Percussive movement, 125, 271
Periodicals, 247
Personal space, 16, 103
Poems and songs, 179-181
Poems
      "A Strong Dance," 128
      "Contrasts in Space," 106-107
      "Contrasts in Time and Space (Elf to Giant)," 98
      "Do Not Bump," 53
      "Four Little Birdies," 185
      "I See the Wind," 184
      "Little Shadow," 183
      "Magic Feet," 184-185
      "Scarf Dance," 160
      "Seeds in the Ground," 186
      "Slow Motion in Weights," 138
      "Snowflakes," 186
      "The Colored Scarf," 159
      "Walking in Space," 121
      "Wings of a Bird," 185
Poetry and props, 159-160
Props, 143-155
Publishers, 238
Pulling, 18
Pushing, 18

Q

R

U

Uneven rhythmic patterns, 19-20

V

Values of creative movement, 9
Vibratory movement, 126, 164
Videos of dance, 239-241

W

Walking, 19
Warm-ups, 26
Warm-up activitives:
    The Body:
        lesson one, 47-54
        lesson two, 64-68
    Time:
        lesson one, 82-83
        lesson two, 88-89
    Space:
        lesson one, 106-108
        lesson two, 115
    Force
        lesson one, 126
        lesson two, 131
    other warm-up activities, 196
Word actions, 188-189
Word ideas, 190-191
Words, 187-190
    body words, 74
    force words, 137
    space words, 120
    time words, 97

AUTHOR INDEX

Ayob, Salmah, 9,

Bennett, John, & Riemer Pamela Coughenour, 222-223,

Boorman, Joyce, 188-189,

Brooks, Nancy, 144,

Dance Grades K-12. A Guide for Idaho Public Schools, 4-5,

Dance as Education, 5, 233

Dorien, Margery, 187, 233

Dunkin, Anne, 3, 233

Fleming, Gladys Andrews, 3, 7, 41, 185-186, 198-199

Gardner, Howard, 6

Gilbert, Anne Green, 2, 219-221

Graham, George, Holt/Hale, Shirley Ann, & Parker, Melissa, 41

Hall, J. Tillman, Sweeny, Nancy Hall, & Esser, Jody Hall, 217-218

Howe, Dianne, & Kimball, Mary Maitland, 230

Humphrey, James, 3

Joyce, Mary, 2, 10, 13, 15, 17, 29, 37, 223-224

Laban, Rudolf, 162

Mettler, Barbara, 190

Mirus, Judith, & White, Elena, 224-225

Mirus, Judith, & White, Elena, & Bucek, Loren, 218, 224, 225-227

Murray, Ruth Lovell, 3, 4

Nash, Grace, 53, 98, 121, 128, 137-139, 159, 160, 179, 186, 199-201

National Standards for Arts Education, 227-230

National Standards for Arts Education. Summary Statement, 227-228

Pre-School Curriculum Guidelines for Malaysia, 8

Purcell, Theresa, 6, 205, 207, 210, 220, 221

Raftis, Alkis, 187

Riggs, Maida, 120, 137

Russell, Joan, 25

Seefeldt, Vern, 120

Stinson, Susan, 10, 218-219

Sullivan, Molly, 36

Tobias, Anne, 11

Wall, Jennifer, & Murray, Nancy, 222

Warren, Jean, 75, 160, 181-185, 197

Waterman, Elizabeth, 164-165

Weikert, Phyllis, 177-178

Zirulnik, Ann, 76

ISBN 9798504074405

9 798504 074405